ABOUT THE AUTHORS

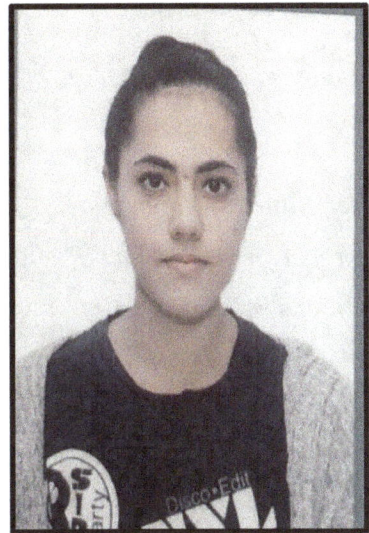

DR. MISCHEAL KAUR SAWHNEY
BDS
MDS FINAL-YEAR POSTGRADUATE
DEPT. OF CONSERVATIVE DENTISTRY AND ENDODONTICS
HIMACHAL DENTAL COLLEGE
SUNDERNAGAR
HIMACHAL PRADESH

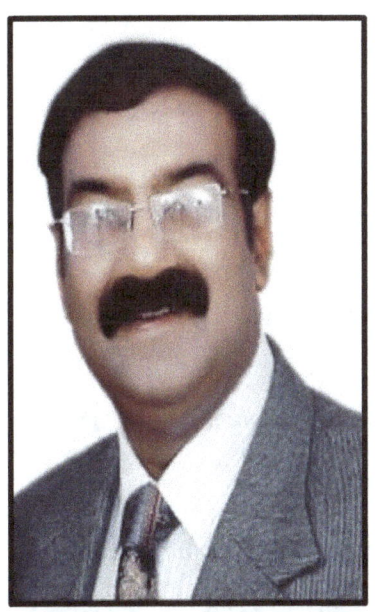

DR. MUNISH GOEL
BDS
MDS
PROFESSOR AND HEAD
DEPT. OF CONSERVATIVE DENTISTRY AND ENDODONTICS
HIMACHAL DENTAL COLLEGE
SUNDERNAGAR
HIMACHAL PRADESH

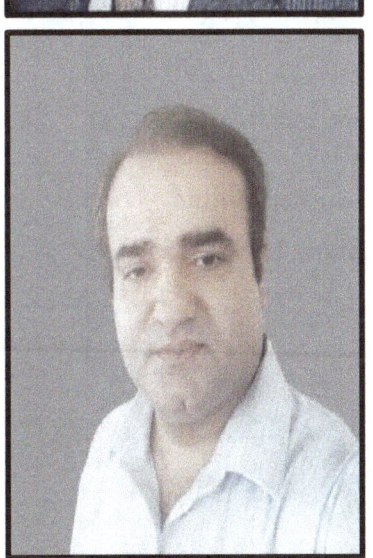

DR. NEERAJ SHARMA
BDS
MDS
PROFESSOR
DEPT. OF CONSERVATIVE DENTISTRY AND ENDODONTICS
HIMACHAL DENTAL COLLEGE
SUNDERNAGAR
HIMACHAL PRADESH

ACKNOWLEDGEMENT

*I offer my fervent prayers and gratitude to **Almighty God** for the blessings showered on me and guiding through every step.*

*I dedicate my profound sense of gratitude to my parents, **Mrs. Satinder Kaur Sawhney** and Late. **Mr. Devinder Singh Sawhney**, for their encouragement, love, great sacrifices, and innate confidence, without which I wouldn't have been where I am today. I am eternally grateful to them for all that they have done for me, without which I would not have been in this position. I owe everything to them. I am extremely fortunate to have an ever-encouraging brother and sister-in-law, **Dr. Jaskaran Singh Sawhney** and **Dr. Manveen Kaur Sawhney** who were my constant pillars and encouraged me to successfully complete this work.*

*Though language is a poor substitute for sentiments, yet there is no way out other than to recourse to it to express my deep respect, sincere gratitude, and regard towards my professor and guide, **Dr. Munish Goel**, MDS, Head of the department, Department of Conservative Dentistry & Endodontics, a great mentor who has always been a source of inspiration to me. I sincerely thank sir for all your painstaking efforts, constant encouragement, constructive suggestions, timely help, fatherly care, and valuable guidance in all my endeavors, bringing out the best in my work. He has always been very understanding, sympathetic, and a great source of support. I cannot emphasize enough how fortunate I feel to work under such an esteemed academician and clinician of outstanding status and experience. I sincerely thank him, for his relentless support, understanding, and dedication.*

*I express my gratitude and everlasting obligation to my co-guide **Dr. Neeraj Sharma**, MDS, Professor, Department of Conservative Dentistry & Endodontics for his extreme patience, invaluable guidance, encouragement, constructive criticism, wise counseling, and painstaking attention to detail during library dissertation work and support throughout this assignment.*

*I deeply express my sincere thanks to **Dr. Vijay Kumar**, MDS, Professor, **Dr. Shweta Verma**, MDS, Professor, **Dr. Kulwant Rai**, MDS, Professor and **Dr. Shilpa Kumari**, MDS, Reader who were always accessible with their words of encouragement and advice which helped me throughout.*

I would also like to extend my sincere gratitude and thanks to **Dr. Anil Singla**, *Director, Himachal Dental College and Hospital, Sundernagar,* **Dr. Vikas Jindal**, *Director, Himachal Dental College and Hospital, Sundernagar, and* **Dr. Baljeet Singh**, *Principal, Himachal Dental College and Hospital, Sundernagar, Himachal Pradesh who made all the facilities available in the institute and also for their continuous support, help, and encouragement to accomplish my assignment.*

I am extremely thankful to my ever-supporting colleagues **Dr. Balkaran, Dr. Jagriti, Dr. Siddhant,** *and* **Dr. Vikrant** *for their support and help. I sincerely thank my seniors* **Dr. Ankush, Dr. Sadaf, Dr. Akshay, Dr. Aryaman,** *and* **Dr. Deepakshi** *who advised and encouraged me throughout this assignment. I would also like to thank my juniors* **Dr. Ashwini, Dr. Shreya, Dr. Shobhita, Dr. Yanger,** *and* **Dr. Diksha** *for being there whenever I needed them.*

A special thanks to **Ms. Harsh, Mr. Kavya, Dr. Ashwini, Dr. Ankush, Dr. Aishwarya, Dr. Ravi, Dr. Nidhisha, Mr. Sahil, Mr. Arshmeet, Dr. Ragini, Mr. Navnish,** *and* **Mr. Pratham** *as this assignment would not have been possible without their help and constant motivation.*

I would like to thank department attendants **Mr. Rattan, Mr. Jagatpal,** *and* **Mrs. Bhawna** *for rendering their timely help throughout my assignment.*

Finally, I would like to thank everybody important to the successful realization of this assignment and I sincerely apologize to those people whose names would have inadvertently slipped my memory.

Dr. Mischeal Kaur Sawhney

CHAPTER-1
INTRODUCTION

The dental profession has devoted most of its history to restoring the effects of dental disease. The last two decades have evidenced a paradigm shift in this philosophy that has been guided by a greater understanding of science. During this evolution, restorative dentistry has adopted a medical model for decision-making in the treatment of dental disease that allows clinicians to individualize and evaluate all components of the process for a proper treatment strategy, including educating and involving the patient in treatment decisions, which results in acceptance of appropriate preventive and restorative strategies and improved compliance and oral health.

The public's interest in health and beauty has become an engine that continues to drive the demand for cosmetic dental procedures. In the past, achieving a beautiful smile required submission to extensive invasive procedures and expensive fixed dental prosthetic restorations. Advancements have expanded the treatment possibilities for the clinician and technician.

Mosby's Dental Dictionary defines esthetic dentistry as, "the skills and techniques used to improve the art and symmetry of the teeth and face to enhance the appearance as well as the function of the teeth, oral cavity, and face." [1] Dental esthetics connects with the principal aspect of appearance—physical attractiveness. Accordingly, esthetic dentistry provides benefits that extend far beyond total dental health toward total well-being throughout life. Esthetics is not absolute, but extremely subjective.

"Many factors and dimensions determine a person's appearance, among which physical attractiveness predominates and which esthetic dentistry can affect favourably. The entirety of the physical attractiveness aspect of appearance calls for the label, physical attractiveness phenomenon."

Gordon Patzer

Notions that esthetic dentistry is only about vanity and caters exclusively to the rich and famous, fail tests of reality. Dental professionals who provide esthetic dentistry and recipients of these services readily offer evidence contrary to this. Functionality matters tremendously. But coupling function with the form improves appearance matters even more.

Rather, it is about the realization that esthetic dentistry done well can contribute to the lives of all people in all walks of life far beyond the in-office, oral cavity, and dental treatment received. Dental esthetics exert a key role in a person's looks, it influences internal self-image, confidence, individual happiness, and external concerning what others see. In other words, it contributes to total dental health and a person's ability to retain or enhance the appearance of his or her teeth contributes accordingly to the world's interactions with that person and vice versa.

HISTORICAL PERSPECTIVE OF DENTAL ESTHETICS

Cosmetic dental treatment dates back more than four millennia. There are repeated references in history to the value of replacing missing teeth. In the El Gigel cemetery near the great Egyptian pyramids, two molars encircled with gold wire were found. Gold was also used to splint anterior teeth and may be thought of as a luxurious way of saving teeth. This was one of the first pieces of evidence showing the Etruscan culture valued the smile as an important part of physical attractiveness. It was a prosthetic device.[2] In the Talmudic Law of the Hebrews, tooth replacement is permitted for women. The Etruscans were well versed in the use of human teeth or teeth carved from animal teeth to restore missing dentition.[3]

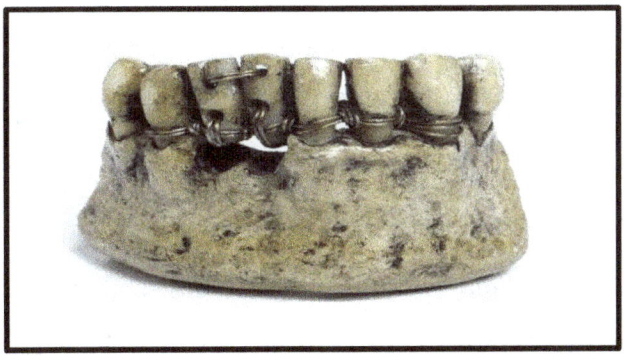

FIGURE 1.1: Over 4000 years ago, the ETRUSCANS demonstrated the earliest treatment related to esthetic dentistry by using gold wire to save diseased teeth to maintain the beauty of the smile. This reproduction shows copper wire. Figure courtesy of the Royal College of Surgeons of Edinburgh.

Other historical evidence of cosmetic alteration of the teeth includes reference to the Japanese custom of decorative tooth-staining called **Ohaguro** in 4000-year-old documents. Described as a purely cosmetic treatment, the procedure had its own set of implements, kept as a cosmetic kit. The chief result of the process was a dark brown or black stain on the teeth. Studies suggest that it might also have had a caries-preventive effect.[4]

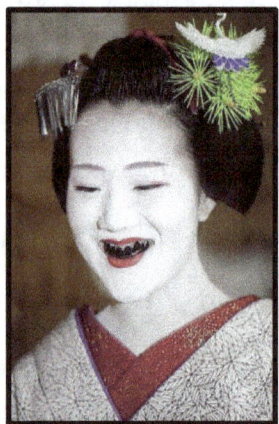
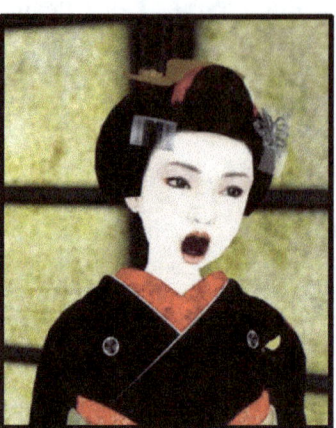

FIGURE 1. 2: Dental esthetics practiced from ancient times in Japan, around 500 A.D, called OHAGURO, in which people stained their teeth to be black in color. This practice continued into the Meiji era, which ended in the early 20th century. Figure courtesy of Dr. Peter Brown.

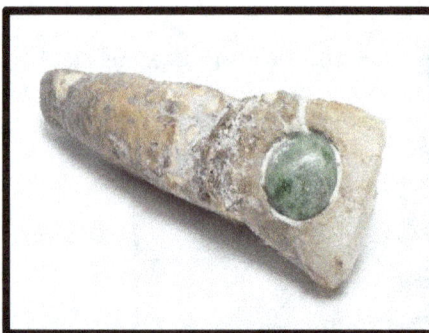
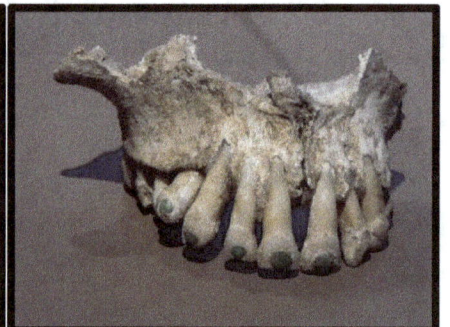

FIGURE 1.3: This 2000-year-old Mayan skull provides some of the best evidence that jadeite inlays were used for cosmetic, rather than functional, purposes. Aside from jadeite inlays, the Mayans also valued using special tooth carvings to enhance physical appearance.[5]

THE SOCIAL CONTEXT OF DENTAL ESTHETICS

In an economically, socially, and sexually competitive world, a pleasing appearance is a necessity. In today's technology-driven society, social media contributes to a person's image being viewed more than ever. As a result, more and more people are considering esthetic dentistry as a necessity to maintain an appealing look. In India **Goleman and Goleman**[6] reported that researchers found that attractive people win more prestigious and higher-paying jobs. They also found that good-looking criminals were less likely to be caught; if they did go to court, they were treated more leniently. Teachers were found to go easier when disciplining attractive children; both teachers and pupils consider attractive children as smarter, nicer, and more apt to succeed at all things. Many studies on self-esteem have illustrated that body image was one of the primary elements in self-rejection.[3-7]

Esthetic dentistry demands attention to the patient's desires and treatment of the patient's problems. Esthetic dentistry is the art of dentistry in its purest form. The purpose is not to sacrifice function but to use it as the foundation of esthetics.

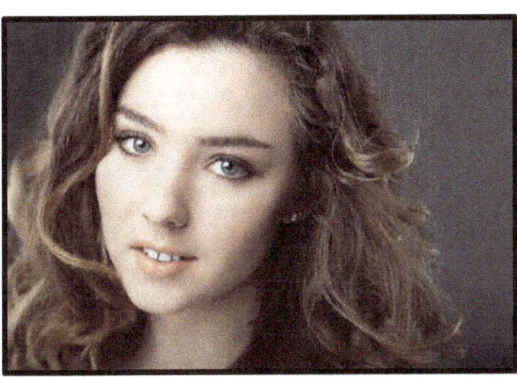 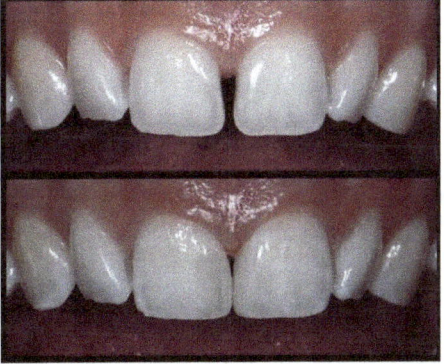

FIGURE 1.4: (a) Image depicting a young girl comfortable with a diastema, and finds it natural, cute, and part of her individuality. (b) Image depicting a case of diastema closure which brings about a new sense of self-confidence and a much more appealing smile was the result of the direct anterior composite restoration. The teeth appear much straighter, brightening the smile and enhances the beauty of her face and lips.

Occasionally, patients take extreme measures to call attention to the mouth in an attempt to achieve an attractive Therefore, it is the responsibility of the dentist to understand what the patient means when using a particular term, and to decide to what degree the patient's ideal may be realized. The patient's feeling of esthetics and concept of self-image are most important.

ESTHETICS: A HEALTH SCIENCE AND SERVICE

Is esthetic dentistry a health science and a health service?[7] Or is it the epitome of vanity working its way into a superficial society?

INTRODUCTION

The answer to these questions lies in the scientific facts gleaned from over a thousand studies proving the direct and indirect relationship of how looking one's best is a key ingredient to a positive self-image, which in turn relates to good mental health. The authors of a survey of nearly 30,000 people point to a relationship between psychosocial well-being and body image.8 They found that feeling attractive, fit, and healthy results in fewer feelings of depression, loneliness, and worthlessness. This study also found that the earlier in life appearance is improved, the more likely it is that the person will go through life with a positive self-image. Sheets states that "An impaired self-image may be more disabling developmentally than the pertinent physical defect."[9] According to Patzer, the face is the most important part of the body when determining physical attractiveness.[10] Specifically, "the hierarchy of importance for facial components appears to be mouth, eyes, facial structure, hair, and nose". Therefore, it becomes apparent that not only should esthetic dentistry be performed but it should also be performed as early as possible.

	RANK ORDER RATINGS BY SELF METHOD		RATINGS BY OTHERS METHOD	
			DISSECTES PHOTOS	INTACT PHOTOS
MOUTH	1	r=0.53	r=0.53	r=0.72
EYES	2	r=0.51	r=0.44	r=0.68
HAIR	3	r=0.49	r=0.34	Not assessed
NOSE	4	r=0.47	r=0.31	r=0.61

Table 1.1 Numerical Ranking of Relative Importance of Face Components Using Three Different Research Methodologies

UNDERSTANDING THE PATIENT'S ESTHETIC NEEDS

A practicing dentist needs to be acquainted with certain generalities concerning the psychological significance of the patient's mouth. He or she should be familiar with basic considerations that apply to esthetic treatment as well as be aware of various problems that such treatments may incur. To be better equipped to anticipate any such problems, a better understanding of physical attractiveness phenomenon is essential.

INTRODUCTION

Physical attractiveness phenomenon

Physical attractiveness is how pleasing someone or something looks. It is a reality perceived. And, as in nearly all of life, perception is more important than reality. However, given its esthetic essence, and its variable/invariable nature constituted by tangibles and intangibles, the perception of physical attractiveness is physical attractiveness. Levels and descriptors range from low or extremely low to high or extremely high physical attractiveness, from very physically unattractive to very physically attractive, and so on.

Its basic definition applies equally to words used interchangeably—beauty, handsomeness, good looks, ugliness, cuteness, and so forth—as well as words used tangentially that express level and polarity such as gorgeous, stunning, head-turner, hunk, hot, voluptuous, pretty, homely dog, pretty ugly. Although both men and women can be judged physically attractive with or without a great smile. However, there are definite attributes to the smile that can enhance one's attractiveness. Teeth add to or subtract from these desired appearances due to their prominent and inescapable presence.

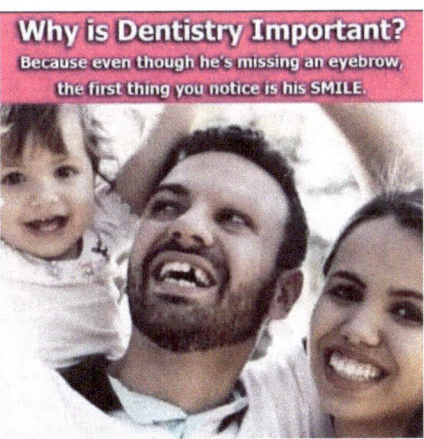

FIGURE 1.5: Image depicting the importance of teeth

Following the eyes' attention to a person's teeth, framed by moving actions of the mouth, people rightfully or wrongly infer far more information about the person observed. Accordingly, teeth considered to look esthetically appealing tend to be accompanied by corresponding inferences, assumptions, stereotypes, and expectations about individuals whose teeth communicate good and positive, bad and negative, or somewhere in between.

The importance of facial appearance

Allport observes, "Most modern research has been devoted not to what the face reveals, but what people think it reveals."[11] He describes tendencies to perceive smiling faces as more intelligent and to see faces that are average in size of the nose, hair, grooming, set of the jaw, and so on, as having more favorable traits than those that deviate from the average. Summarizing an experiment by Brunswick and Reiter, Allport notes, "One finding…is that in general, the mouth is the most decisive facial feature in shaping our judgments."[4] Studies suggest that even infants can tell an attractive face when they see one, long before they learn society's standards for beauty. Results of experiments with two groups of infants were reported by psychologist Judith Langlois and five colleagues at the University of Texas at Austin. Seventy-one percent of the infants looked longer at attractive faces than at unattractive faces.[12-16]

Functions Of Teeth

The appearance of a person's teeth communicates much about that person. Therefore, it is not surprising what people can actually achieve with their teeth and smiles. The functions of teeth in the minds of many people include the role of communicating information. Part of the way we communicate is through smiling at one another. Proper functioning of teeth for these people means more than chewing well and pain-free. They believe consciously or subconsciously that the look of their teeth substantially influences the perception of themselves by themselves and by others. Demeaning comments, shunning, and even bullying becomes a way of living for individuals sentenced to visibly missing, crowded, spaced, or protrusive teeth, or other dental anomalies. This is true at least for those individuals without the means for corrective action toward fewer negative appearances of their teeth. These individuals make ill-fated attempts to avoid those negative reactions. Typical attempts include avoiding all smiling for fear of showing their esthetically unappealing teeth, concocting a smile that never shows teeth, or using a hand or napkin to cover the mouth while speaking face to face. Tolls on a person can be particularly great on those of younger ages. The negative consequences go far beyond affecting only self-image and self-confidence. The mouth can be a particularly significant component of a person's physical attractiveness, which at the same time is rather inseparable from teeth and a smile. One of psychology's most revered, Gordon Allport, once observed that people perceive smiling faces to be more intelligent[11] and, citing another research project noted, "…in general the mouth is the most decisive facial feature in shaping our judgments" about a person.[2] An improved self-image leading to increased self-confidence with assistance from esthetic dentistry is not limited to teenage girls. A good smile in these regards can produce improvements in psychological and social well-being for individuals of all ages in all walks of life.

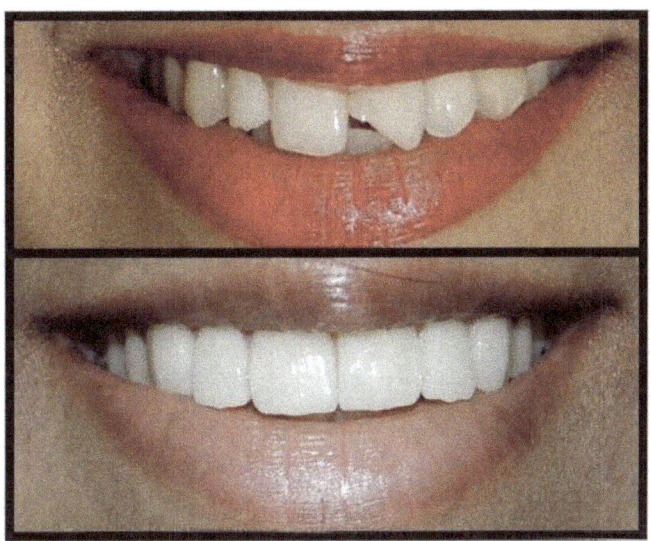

FIGURE 1.6: Image of a case of Ellis class II fracture repaired with a ceramic crown which helped the patient gain a new sense of self-confidence after cosmetic dentistry transformed her unpleasing smile into a much more appealing smile.

Patient Response to Abnormality

The smile is the baby's most regularly evoked response and eventually signifies pleasure. Thus, any aberration it reveals can naturally be a point of anxiety. Abnormality implies difference, a characteristic undesirable to most people. However, as **Rottersman** notes, "The response may not be out of all proportion to the stimulus. This is a signal for the doctor to exercise caution, and to attempt to discern what truly underlies the patient's response" (**W. Rottersman**, personal communication). Understanding the patient's motives requires acute perception on the dentist's part, informed by a thorough examination and history that reveal the patient's actual dental problems.[17] The patient's own assessment of his problems and his reaction to them are of equal importance. The dentist should be alert for displacement syndrome, in which anxiety aroused by real and major emotional problems may be transferred to a minor oral deformity. When a patient with a long-standing complaint finally presents for treatment, the dentist must determine what prevented him or her from coming for treatment sooner. A patient who criticizes a former dentist is apt to be hostile, and the dentist should not present a treatment plan before determining what the patient believes the treatment can accomplish.

Patient types and dentist alerts

The reasons why patients seek esthetic treatment are as varied and intricate as the reasons they avoid it. How adults feel about and care for their mouths often reflects past, current, and future oral developmental experiences. Adults in their mid-20s may not have developed a sense of the meaning of time in the life cycle. Lack of oral health care may reflect a denial of mortality and normal body degeneration. Between the ages of 35 and 40 adults become reconciled to the fact they are aging and a renewed interest in self-preservation emerges. This interest is often directed toward various types of self-improvements such as orthodontic, cosmetic restorative, cosmetic periodontal, plastic or orthognathic surgery, or any combination of these.

Burns, in his discussion of motivations for orthodontic treatment, cites the results of a study by **Jarabak** who determined five stimuli that may move a patient toward orthodontia. The motives, also applicable to esthetic dentistry, are as follows:

(1) social acceptance, (2) fear, (3) intellectual acceptance, (4) personal pride, and (5) biological benefits. (It should be noted that these stimuli pertain only to patients who cooperate in treatment.)[7,18]

Much psychological theory in dental esthetics must be formulated through analogy because of the comparatively recent recognition of the importance of dental esthetics and the consequent lack of a comprehensive database. The most obvious parallel field is plastic surgery. In a pioneering paper published in 1939, **Baker and Smith**[19, 21] posited a system that categorized 312 patients into three groups based on personality traits:

Group I—Ideal individuals for successful treatment with well-adjusted personalities, moderate success in life, aware that all life problems cannot be solved by better-looking teeth, and realistically want treatment to improve esthetics and/or for greater comfort. They want repair of their disfigurements for cosmetic reasons or comfort, not as an answer to all their problems. They do not expect too much from the improvement and they have a realistic visual concept of the outcome. They are ideal subjects for successful treatment.

Group II—Irksome individuals of two types. The very irksome type are individuals who remain unhappy with results despite the excellent technical outcome achieved through prior treatment, indicating the same will happen with future treatments. Underlying that unhappiness, they continue past dysfunctional thinking about their prior appearance defects causing unrelated life problems outside the oral cavity or they find actual life with better-looking teeth to be not as great as they had earlier unrealistically fantasized.

A substantially less irksome type in this Group II category are passive apologetic individuals who are grateful for any and all treatment, even though past results proved technically unsatisfactory as likely will be results of future treatments.

Group III—Individuals with psychotic personalities for whom treatment outcomes will never be satisfactory in their view, regardless of actual technical results. Their visibly unattractive dental esthetics that existed before treatment served them as a focal point of their life problems and will probably continue always. Soon, some other defect is seized upon as the focus for their continuing psychotic delusions. These individuals warrant other professional treatment such as psychological or psychiatric counselling because dental treatment alone likely only disrupts their delusional rationalizations with no significant benefit in the longer term.

As expressed above, patients focused on cosmetic dentistry can be greatly appreciative and/or greatly demanding. Nevertheless, they must all be satisfied with their results.

Advanced measures, pre-treatment, by the dentist to improve the likelihood of post-treatment satisfaction include the following:

● Listen well to the wants and perspectives of the patient before embarking on treatment. This "listening" extends to observing well any possible pertinent nonverbal clues exhibited by the patient.

● Discuss well any concerns, questions, expectations, and as much or little detail as appropriate for the individual patient.

● Present treatment options along with their procedures, timelines, advantages, and disadvantages or limitations.

- Be "realistically idealistic," expressing the ideal but realistic scenario while being neither unrealistically optimistic that then builds too high of expectations that cannot be met and will generate dissatisfaction.

- Trial smile procedures, discussed in later chapters.

REFERENCES

1. **Aboucaya WA**. The Dento-Labial Smile and the Beauty of the Face [thesis]. No. 50. Academy of Paris, University of Paris VI; 1973.

2. **Anderson JN.** The value of teeth. Br Dent J 1965; 119:98.

3. **Guerini V.** A History of Dentistry from the Most Ancient Times Until the End of the Eighteenth Century. New York: Milford House; 1969.

4. **Ai S, Ishikawa T.** "Ohaguro" traditional tooth staining custom in Japan. Int Dent J 1965.

5. https://anthropology.net/2007/06/01/damien-hirsts-diamondencrusted-skull-jeweled-skulls-in-archaeology/.

6. **Goleman D, Goleman TB**. Beauty's hidden equation. Am Health [now the Time-Warner publication Health]. March 1987.

7. **Jarabak JR.** Management of an Orthodontic Practice. St. Louis, MO: CV Mosby; 1956.

8. **Cash TF, Winstead BA, Janda LH.** The great American shaped up. Psychol Today 1986:30–37.

9. **Sheets CG.** Modern dentistry and the esthetically aware patient. J Am Dent Assoc 1987:115:103E–105E.

10. **Patzer GL.** Looks: Why They Matter More Than You Ever Imagined. New York: AMACOM Books; 2008.

11. **Allport GW.** Pattern and Growth in Personality. New York: Holt and Rinehart; 1961:479.

12. **Langlois JH.** Attractive faces get the attention of infants. Atlanta Journal 1987; May 6:6.

13. **Langlois JH.** From the eye of the beholder to behavioral reality: the development of social behaviors and social relations as a function of physical attractiveness. In: Herman CP, Zanna MP, Higgins ET, eds. Physical Appearance, Stigma, and Social Behavior: The Ontario Symposium. Hillsdale, NJ: Erlbaum; 1986:23–51.

14. **Langlois JH, Roggman LA.** Attractive faces are only average. Am Psychol Soc 1990; 1:115–121.

15. **Langlois JH, Roggman LS, Casey RJ, et al.** Infant preferences for attractive faces: rudiments of a stereotype? Dev Psychol 1987; 23:363–369. 18.

16. **Langlois JH, Roggman LA, Rieser-Danner LA.** Infant's differential social responses to attractive and unattractive faces. Dev Psychol 1990;26(1):153–159.
17. **Levinson N.** Psychological facets of esthetic dentistry: a developmental perspective. J Prosthet Dent 1990; 64:486–491.
18. **Burns MH.** Use of a personality rating scale in identifying cooperative and non-cooperative orthodontic patients. Am J Orthod 1970; 57:418.
19. **Baker WY, Smith LH.** Facial disfigurement and personality. JAMA 1939; 112:301.

CHAPTER-2
DIAGNOSTICS AND SHADE MATCHING

Excellence will never be achieved by chance, but by using a consistent systematic approach for diagnosis, communication, treatment planning, and execution. The incorporation of protocols and checklists [1-7] for quality control and information management will guarantee that every critical point is performed effectively, double-checked, and communicated correctly.

The diagnostic work-up is the foundation of any successful restorative therapy.[8] This phase of treatment planning provides the restorative team (i.e., patient, general dentist, technician, and specialist) with time to evaluate, visualize, and predict the functional and esthetic outcome prior to performing any restorative or surgical procedure. Although time-consuming, this diagnostic approach allows for more predictable results and potential obstacles related to preparation, occlusion, and esthetics to be overcome. This process eliminates misunderstanding among the team members through communication, improved predictability, and chair-time efficiency. Because communication is characteristic of a progressive profession,[9,10] the restorative team must constantly remain knowledgeable in current trends while staying accessible to the colloquy of information between them. A commonality of goals and interests, values, desires, and capabilities represent an important developmental criterion for the team.[11]

Improving each individual's understanding of the other members' contributions may also result in effective interdisciplinary communication.[12] Once the design, materials, techniques, and esthetic concepts are mastered by each team member,[13] a higher standard of dental service can be provided to the patient. There are several communication tools that can be used to effectively transmit information between the restorative team, including photography, shade determination and diagramming, and diagnostic models.

SHADE DETERMINATION

When fabricating a restoration, patient satisfaction with the shade match is essential. The patient's level of satisfaction may not be the same as that of the dental practitioner. Esthetic expectations have dramatically increased in the last few years. Color and shade determination is generally considered difficult in dental practice. However, owing to the extensive range of natural tooth colors, achieving an intimate shade match between the prosthesis and natural teeth is challenging. The human brain can identify nearly one million shades, and precise devices that can recognize approximately 10 million different shades have been developed. Human dentition shades differ significantly, and electronic devices can identify approximately 100,000 dental shades while the human eye can identify only 1% of these shades.[14]

It is difficult to accurately describe and verbally communicate shades; hence, three variables are used to characterize the perception of light reflected from the tooth surface: **hue, value, and chroma**.

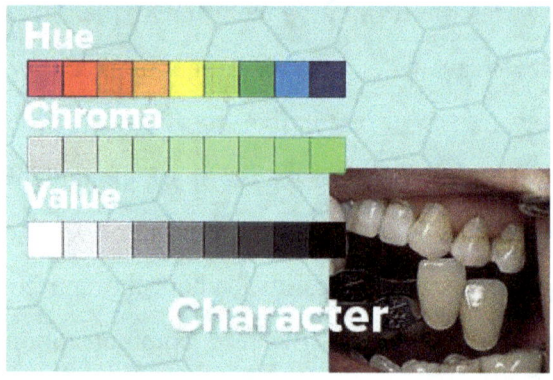

FIGURE 2.1: HUE, CHROMA, VALUE

Hue describes the dominant shade of the tooth (more yellowish or reddish), value is the lightness or darkness of the tooth shade measured independently of the hue, and chroma is the quality that distinguishes the degree of vividness of the hue.[15]

Shade-matching devices are also called shade guides. The order of shade selection is first selecting the value, chroma, and lastly hue. Color matching should be done in a systematic way that ensures accuracy, uniformity, and predictable results which are absolutely important in esthetic dentistry.

Operating Site Lighting

Sunlight in the middle of the day is considered optimal for shade selection, as this exposure contains an almost equal blend of all wavelengths of light compared to morning and evening exposures, which are richer in reddish and yellow wavelengths. In clinics that do not have proper access to sunlight, artificial light should be used to simulate sunlight. Although no artificial light lamp can perfectly duplicate sunlight, it is adequate for clinical purposes. Prior to shade selection, the light to which the patients are most exposed in their daily routine must be ascertained.[14,15-17]

Environment

Bright-colored surroundings should be avoided as they interfere with proper color matching by influencing the colors in the reflected light. A drape can be used to mask undesirable colors in the patient's clothing and jewellery. Lipstick should be removed so that it does not affect color perception. A very light grey color provides the ideal background for color matching. Surfaces with high gloss produce disturbing glares and should be avoided.[14,15-17]

Condition of the Teeth

The tooth of interest and its adjacent teeth should be free of plaque and other deposits and surface stains. The tooth should be moist with saliva as dehydration results in a whiter appearance. The tooth becomes dryer after the application of the rubber dam, and therefore, color matching should be performed before applying it.[14,15-17]

Distance of the Operator from the Tooth, Position of the Patient, and Timing

A distance of 61 cm (2 feet) to 183 cm (6 feet) distance from the oral cavity is considered ideal for shade matching.[14,15-17] The patient should be positioned in the dental chair such that the patient's teeth are at the level of the operator's eyes. The operator should stand directly in front of the patient, with light focused on the teeth.[14,15-17] Shade selection and shade matching should be performed by the dentist preferably in the morning when eye fatigue is minimal.[14,15-17]

Squint Test for Restricting Light

The squint test enables shade selection by restricting the light entering the eye. It is performed by bringing the eyelids closer and then looking at the shade guide and the natural tooth. The color that fades from view first is the one that is least conspicuous in comparison with the tooth color.[18] There are two types of shade selection methods: the conventional method and the use of color-measuring instruments.[14]

Visual shade guides

The conventional method of shade selection is the use of visual shade guides which are the most popular and convenient way of selecting tooth shades. They are cost-effective and readily available; they also proficiently match the color of the dentition with a standardized reference shade guide. The selection of tooth color by the shade tab method completely depends on human eye observation. The currently available shade tabs are Vita classical (Bad Säckingen, Germany: VITA Zahnfabrik H. Rauter GmbH & Co.), Vita Toothguide 3D-Master shade guide (Bad Säckingen, Germany: VITA Zahnfabrik H. Rauter GmbH & Co.), and Chromascop (Buffalo, NY: Ivoclar Vivadent Inc.).[19]

Vita Classical Shade Guide

Based on the hue, 16 tabs are arranged into four groups and within the groups corresponding to the chroma. Since there are some limitations with Vita classical shade guide, the Vita 3D-Master shade guide is the most commonly used among the commercially available shade tabs. It provides superior and standardized colour differences.[20,21]

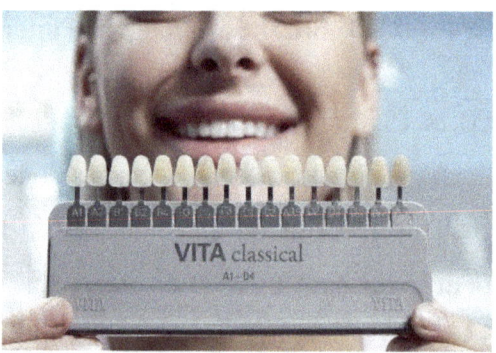

FIGURE 2.2: VITA CLASSICAL SHADE GUIDE

Vita Toothguide 3D-Master

It comprises 26 tabs separated into five groups depending on the lightness of the color. The numbers (1, 2, 3, 4, and 5) in front of the letters represent the group number and lightness level; a lower number indicates a higher lightness. The numbers (1, 1.5, 2, 2.5, and 3) below the group number represent the level of the chroma; the more chromatic tabs are indicated by larger numbers. Three bleaching shades (0M1, 0M2, and 0M3) indicate more lightness, three levels of chroma, and a middle hue. The major contrast between the Vita Classical and Vita 3D-Master is that the Vita Classical shade guide is built on the colour hue and the Vita 3D-Master characterizes the colour value. The Vita 3D-Master shade guide is considered superior to the Vita classical shade guide. It contains enhanced lightness spectrum and additional chromatic tabs. The hue latitude is expanded against the reddish spectra. Further, the shade tabs are evenly distributed and group division is improved.[22-24]

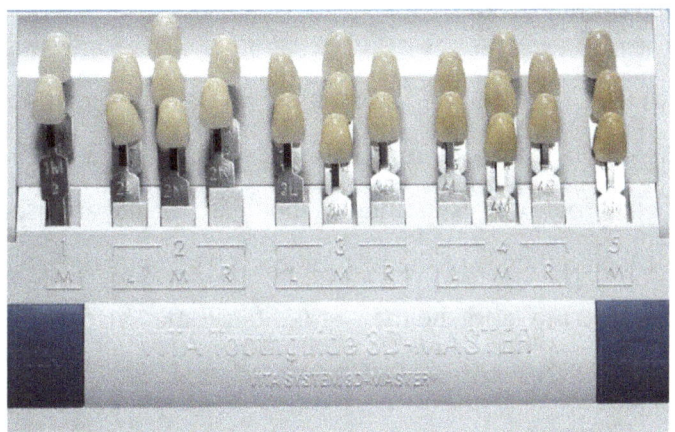

FIGURE 2.3: VITA TOOTH GUIDE 3-D MASTER

Chromascop

Chromascop uses a numbering system to identify shades. It is organized into groups depending on the hue (100 = white, 200 = yellow, 300 = orange, 400 = gray, 500 = brown) and within the groups as chroma increases from 10 to 40.[16]

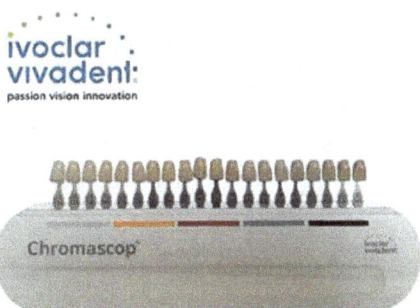

FIGURE 2.4: CHROMASCOP

Custom Shade Guides

The standard shade guide cannot encompass the entire range of hue and chroma values of human dentition. It is useful for 85% of the color selection, and its alteration or preparation of custom shade tabs is necessary for the remaining 15%. Composite resin, ceramic, or acrylic materials are used to fabricate custom-made shade guides. Shade guide modifications can be performed using surface colorants or by surface abrasion using aluminum oxide. Fine line markers and colored pencils may be used to reproduce the minute variations between shades, analogous translucency, and denominating colors.[25]

Dentin and Extended Shade Guides

The dentin system can be used for the fabrication of translucent all-ceramic crowns and veneers. This shade guide helps in communicating a specific shade to the dental laboratory. Specially colored die materials corresponding to the dentin shade are used, which allows the technician to appraise the aesthetics of the restoration.[26] The extended shade guide comprises the tabs of all materials used to fabricate the restoration. It may also be utilized to expand the choice of shade.[27]

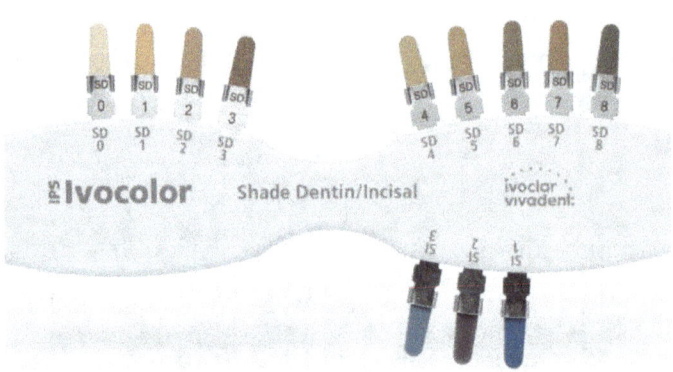

FIGURE 2.5: IVOCLAR IPS EMPRESS DENTIN/INCISAL SHADE GUIDE

Disadvantages of shade guides

The disadvantages of shade guides are described as follows:

(a) the colors in shade guides differ for each manufacturing company;

(b) porcelain used for restoration may not be identical to that used in a guide;

(c) guides are unable to direct the fabrication of porcelain restorations;

(d) the shades in a guide are not logically organized and do not cover the volume of color space that exists in natural dentition;

(e) a standard shade tab is made using synthetic resin and has greater thickness than that of a crown;

(f) a shade guide tab reflects and transmits light, creating translucency and an appearance of vitality.[28,29]

However, for a restoration, light is reflected and is less likely to be transmitted, which makes the restoration appear dense and opaque.

Color measuring instruments

All color-measuring devices comprise three parts: a detector, signal conditioner, and software that converts the signal into data that can be used in the dental laboratory or operatory. The following are examples of color measuring instruments:

(1) colorimeters,

(2) spectrophotometers,

(3) digital cameras,

(4) hybrid devices, and

(5) spectroradiometers.

Colorimeter

A colorimeter measures color (hue, chroma, and value) as perceived by the human eye. It can only measure color by measuring tristimulus values under fixed illumination and observer conditions. The light source, integrating sphere, and detector (three or four filters) are the key optical elements.[19,28]

Spectrophotometer

Spectrophotometers are commonly used to analyze surface colors. They measure the amount of spectral reflection from the body. It is a photometer that can measure intensity based on color, specifically wavelength. The optical elements consist of a light source, monochromator, and detector. In general, light sources are diffracted. Several wavelengths are passed through the entrance slit and the test sample is tested.[30] Different wavelengths of light are selectively absorbed by the sample. The light then passes through another slit, called the exit slit, and strikes the detector. The detector converts the intensity of light at a certain wavelength into an electrical signal, which is then amplified and displayed on a screen or plotted on a chart. It is advisable to use a spectrophotometer to accurately measure color. A colorimeter provides an overall measure of the light absorbed, while a spectrophotometer measures the light absorbed at varying wavelengths. Briefly, colorimeters measure the amount of light absorbed overall, while spectrophotometers measure the amount of light absorbed by a specific wavelength. Spectrophotometers are reliable and accurate over time.[31]

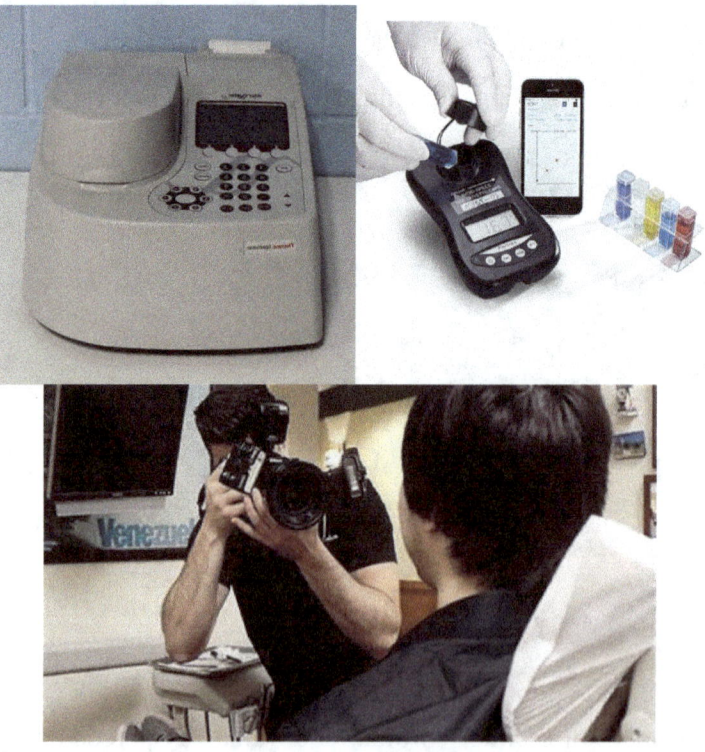

FIGURE 2.6: COLORIMETER, SPECTROPHOTOMETER AND DIGITAL CAMERA

Digital Cameras

A digital camera is the most basic form of an electronic shade-matching device. In contrast to film cameras, this device records images using charge-coupled devices (CCDs), which comprise thousands or even millions of minute light-sensitive elements known as photosites. It provides a thorough and precise picture of the tooth surface and is also useful for color mapping. There is a flashcard that records all memories and allows the recording of voice feedback that can be sent directly to the lab without the need for a computer. The data can be downloaded onto a computer system for easy shade and translucency mapping.[32,33]

Hybrid Devices

SpectroShade provides a combination of digital imaging and spectrophotometric analyses. It uses the ClearMatch software system (Hood River, OR: Smart Technology) and is a hardware-independent product developed for use on all personal computers having the Windows platform and almost any digital camera.[34]

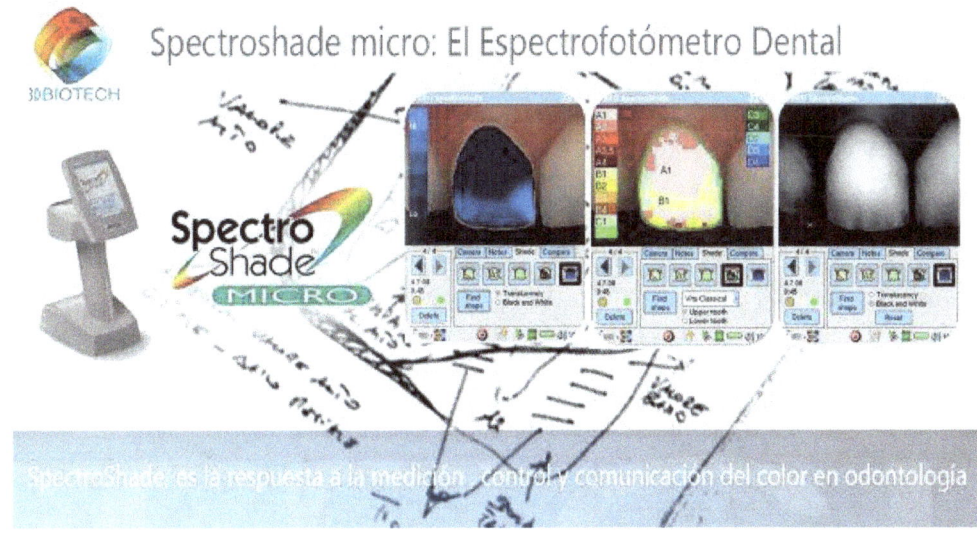

FIGURE 2.7: SPECTROSHADE SOFTWARE SYSTEM

Spectrophotometers and Spectroradiometers

These instruments allow the most precise color measurements. A spectrophotometer differs from a spectroradiometer in that it mainly contains a steady source of light. Two different basic designs have been employed for these instruments. The conventional scanning device comprises a single photodiode detector that records the quantity of light at each wavelength.[35] The latest design utilizes a diode array with a dedicated element for each wavelength. This design allows the simultaneous integration of all wavelengths at the same time. Both designs operate significantly slower than filter colorimeters but remain important for research on the development of precise colour-measuring devices.[36]

Limitations of digital shade guide

The limitations of the digital shade guide include the following:

(a) the phenomenon of edge loss affects the accuracy of color measurement;

(b) translucent mapping is inadequate for all systems;

(c) placement of the probe or mouthpiece seems to be important for the repeatability of the measurement;

(d) no digital shade guide is sufficiently advanced to operate in a formulation mode;

(e) the laboratory must have up-to-date systems for the successful application of this approach; (f) this approach requires a relatively expensive setup.[33, 37]

REFERENCES

1. **Coachman C, Van Dooren E, Gürel G, et al.** Smile design: from digital treatment planning to clinical reality. In: Cohen M, ed. Interdisciplinary Treatment Planning. Vol. II: Comprehensive Case Studies. Hanover Park, IL: Quintessence; 2011.

2. **Goldstein RE.** Esthetics in Dentistry: Principles, Communication, Treatment Methods. Ontario, ON: B. C. Decker; 1998.

3. **Chiche GJ, Pinault A.** Esthetics of Anterior Fixed Prosthodontics. Hanover Park, IL: Quintessence; 1996.

4. **Magne P, Belser U.** Bonded Porcelain Restorations in the Anterior Dentition: A Biomimetic Approach. Carol Stream, IL: Quintessence; 2002.

5. **Fradeani M.** Esthetic Rehabilitation in Fixed Prosthodontics: Esthetic Analysis: A Systematic Approach to Prosthetic Treatment. Carol Stream, IL: Quintessence; 2004.

6. **Gürel G.** The Science and Art of Porcelain Laminate Veneers. Berlin: Quintessence; 2003.

7. **Rufenacht CR.** Fundamentals of Esthetics. Carol Stream, IL: Quintessence; 1990.

8. **Magne P, Belser U.** Bonded Porcelain Restorations in the Anterior Dentition: A Biomimetic Approach. Chicago:Quintessence, 2002.

9. **Ubassy G.** Shape and Color:The Key to Successful Ceramic Restorations Chicago: Quintessence, 1993.

10. **Terry DA, Moreno C, Geller W, Roberts M.** The importance of laboratory communication in modern dental practice: Stone models without faces. Pract Periodontics Aesthet Dent 1999; 11:1 125-1132.

11. **Levin R.** Working with your dental laboratory. Dent Econ 1991; 81:47—50.

12. **Muia P.** Bench talk. Paul Muia explains his four-dimensional tooth color system. Quintes- sence DentTechnol 1983; 7:57-62.

13. **O'Keefe KL, Strickler ER, Kerrin HK.** Color and shade matching: The weak link in esthetic dentistry. Compend Contin Educ Dent 1990; 11:116-120.

14. **Özat PB, Tuncel İ, Eroğlu E**: Repeatability and reliability of human eye in visual shade selection. J Oral Rehabil. 2013, 40:958-64. 10.1111/joor.12103

15. **Basavanna R, Gohil C, Shivanna V**: Shade selection. Int J Oral Health Sci. 2013, 3:26-31. 10.4103/2231-6027.122097

16. **Bhat V, Prasad DK, Sood S, Bhat A**: Role of colors in prosthodontics: application of color science in restorative dentistry. Indian J Dent Res. 2011, 22:804-9. 10.4103/0970-9290.94675
17. **Clark E**: Tooth color selection. J Am Dent Assoc. 1933, 20:1065-73. 10.14219/jada.archive.1933.0149
18. **Sikri VK**: Color: implications in dentistry. J Conserv Dent. 2010, 13:249-55. 10.4103/0972-0707.73381
19. **Sulaiman AO, Adebayo GE**: Most frequently selected shade for advance restoration delivered in a tertiary hospital facility in south western Nigeria. Ann Ib Postgrad Med. 2019, 17:157-61.
20. **Kalantari MH, Ghoraishian SA, Mohaghegh M**: Evaluation of accuracy of shade selection using two spectrophotometer systems: Vita Easyshade and Degudent Shadepilot. Eur J Dent. 2017, 11:196-200. 10.4103/ejd.ejd_195_16
21. **Hombesh MN, Praveen B, Sinha HV, Prasanna BG, Sachin B, Chandrashekar S**: Two years survivability of VITA 3D master shade matching guides after disinfection with isopropyl alcohol: an in vitro study. J Conserv Dent. 2019, 22:275-80. 10.4103/JCD.JCD_573_18
22. **Corcodel N, Rammelsberg P, Jakstat H, Moldovan O, Schwarz S, Hassel AJ**: The linear shade guide design of Vita 3D-master performs as well as the original design of the Vita 3D-master. J Oral Rehabil. 2010, 37:860-5. 10.1111/j.1365-2842.2010.02120.x
23. **Gómez-Polo C, Gómez-Polo M, de Parga JA, Celemín-Viñuela A**: Clinical study of the 3D-master color system among the Spanish population. J Prosthodont. 2018, 27:708-15. 10.1111/jopr.12584
24. **Parameswaran V, Anilkumar S, Lylajam S, Rajesh C, Narayan V**: Comparison of accuracies of an intraoral spectrophotometer and conventional visual method for shade matching using two shade guide systems. J Indian Prosthodont Soc. 2016, 16:352-8. 10.4103/0972-4052.176537
25. **Rajan N, Krishna S R, Rajan A, Singh G, Jindal L**: Shade selection - basic for esthetic dentistry: literature review. Int J Contemp Res Rev. 2020, 11:10.15520/ijcrr.v11i09.849
26. **Fondriest J**: Shade matching in restorative dentistry: the science and strategies. Int J Periodontics Restorative Dent. 2003, 23:467-79.

27. **Paolone G, Orsini G, Manauta J, Devoto W, Putignano A**: Composite shade guides and color matching. Int J Esthet Dent. 2014, 9:164-82.
28. **Todorov R, Yordanov B, Peev T, Zlatev S**: Shade guides used in the dental practice. J of IMAB. 2020, 26:3168-73. 10.5272/jimab.2020262.3168
29. **Joiner A**: Tooth colour: a review of the literature. J Dent. 2004, 32:3-12. 10.1016/j.jdent.2003.10.013
30. **Suganya SP, Manimaran P, Saisadan D, Kumar CD, Abirami D, Monnica V**: Spectrophotometric evaluation of shade selection with digital and visual methods. J Pharm Bioallied Sci. 2020, 12:319-23. 10.4103/jpbs.JPBS_95_20
31. **Ballard E, Metz MJ, Harris BT, Metz CJ, Chou JC, Morton D, Lin WS**: Satisfaction of dental students, faculty, and patients with tooth shade-matching using a spectrophotometer. J Dent Educ. 2017, 81:545-53. 10.21815/JDE.016.022
32. **Wee AG, Lindsey DT, Kuo S, Johnston WM**: Color accuracy of commercial digital cameras for use in dentistry. Dent Mater. 2006, 22:553-9. 10.1016/j.dental.2005.05.011
33. **Jarad FD, Russell MD, Moss BW**: The use of digital imaging for colour matching and communication in restorative dentistry. Br Dent J. 2005, 199:43-9. 10.1038/sj.bdj.4812559
34. **Brewer JD, Wee A, Seghi R**: Advances in color matching. Dent Clin North Am. 2004, 48:341-58. 10.1016/j.cden.2004.01.004
35. **Chu SJ, Trushkowsky RD, Paravina RD**: Dental color matching instruments and systems. Review of clinical and research aspects. J Dent. 2010, 38:2-16. 10.1016/j.jdent.2010.07.001
36. **Miyajiwala JS, Kheur MG, Patankar AH, Lakha TA**: Comparison of photographic and conventional methods for tooth shade selection: a clinical evaluation. J Indian Prosthodont Soc. 2017, 17:273-81. 10.4103/jips.jips_342_16
37. **Bayindir F, Kuo S, Johnston WM, Wee AG**: Coverage error of three conceptually different shade guide systems to vital unrestored dentition. J Prosthet Dent. 2007, 98:175-85. 10.1016/S0022-3913(07)60053-5

CHAPTER-3
DIGITAL SMILE DESIGNING

The Digital Smile Design (DSD) is a practical multiuse clinical tool with relevant advantages: it can strengthen esthetic diagnostic abilities, improve the communication between team members, create predictable systems throughout the treatment phases, enhance the patient's education and motivation, and increase the effectiveness of case presentation. It is an effective digital treatment protocol that utilizes 2-D clinical and lab images of the patient and the proposed treatment plan including planes of reference, facial and dental midlines, incisal edge position, lip dynamics, basic tooth arrangement, and the incisal plane. Digitally drawing reference lines and shapes over the patient's photo, following a predetermined sequence, allows the team to better evaluate the esthetic relation between the teeth, the gingiva, the smile, and the face. DSD is an extraordinary multi-purpose tool that can be utilized by all team members to better understand, visualize, and implement the treatment plan. As the use of the DSD can make the diagnosis more effective and the treatment planning more consistent, the effort required to implement it will be rewarded, making the treatment sequence more logical and straightforward, saving time and materials, and reducing the costs during the treatment.

Advantages of Digital Smile Design

a) **Accurate esthetic analysis**: The DSD allows careful esthetic analysis of the patient's facial and dental features and a gradual discovery of many critical factors that might have been overlooked during the evaluation of clinical, photographic, or study models. The drawing of reference lines and shapes over extra- and intraoral digital photographs performed in presentation software such as Keynote (Apple iWork) or MS Powerpoint (Microsoft Office), following a predetermined sequence, will enhance the diagnostic vision. It also helps the team assess and understand limitations and risk factors such as asymmetries, disharmonies, and violations of esthetic principles, adding critical data to the treatment planning process.[1]

b) **Increased communication among the interdisciplinary team**: The main goal of the DSD protocol is to simplify communication, transferring key information from the patient's face to the working cast, and to the final restoration. It provides effective communication between the interdisciplinary team members, including the dental technician. All team members can access this information whenever necessary— "in the cloud"— changing or adding new elements during the diagnostic and treatment phases. e ability to communicate the patient's personal preferences and/or morpho-psychological features to the laboratory technician, providing information that can elevate the quality of the restoration from one that is adequate to one that is viewed by the patient as exceptional.[2, 3, 4]

c) **Feedback at each phase of treatment**: The DSD allows a precise re-evaluation of the results obtained in every phase of the treatment. The sequence of the treatment is organized on the slides with photos, videos, reports, graphics, and drawings, making this analysis simple and effective. With the Digital Ruler, with which drawings and reference lines are created, it is possible to perform simple comparisons between the before and after pictures, determining if they are in accordance with the original planning, or if any other adjunctive procedures are necessary to improve the outcome. This constant double-checking ensures that a higher-quality product will be delivered from the laboratory and also provides a great learning tool for the entire interdisciplinary team.

d) **Patient understanding and marketing tool**: It is an important marketing tool to motivate the patient, making him or she understand the issues and treatment options, compare before and after pictures, and value all the work that was done. Also, generates a personal library of clinical cases that can be shared with other patients and colleagues, and the most appropriate cases can be further transformed into interesting slideshows of one's work.

e) **Dynamic and effective treatment planning presentation**: It makes the treatment planning presentation more effective and clearer. The case presentation will be more effective and dynamic for these patients since the problem list will be superimposed over their own photographs, increasing the understanding, trust, and acceptance of the proposed plan. The clinician can express the severity of the case, introduce strategies for treatment, discuss the prognosis, and make case management recommendations.[1]

f) **Educational tool**: The DSD can increase the impact of the presentations because it adds visual elements to the slides that will improve the educational aspects of the lecture. The audience can better understand the issues previously highlighted and the presenter can minimize the use of the laser pointer.

DIGITAL SMILE DESIGN WORKFLOW

The DSD protocol is performed by the authors using **Keynote**; however, other similar software such as **MS PowerPoint** can also be used with minor adjustments in the technique. Keynote allows simple manipulation of digital images and the addition of lines, shapes, drawings, and measurements over clinical and laboratory images. The main steps of the DSD are described and illustrated below.

In order to begin the process, three basic photos are necessary: full-face at rest, full-face with a wide smile and teeth apart, and a retracted photo of the upper arch with teeth apart.

A short video is also recommended capturing the following lip positions: at rest, a wide smile stretched from a frontal view, 45°, and profile. In this video, a few basic questions can be asked of the patient to explain their main concerns, needs, and expectations. Then, the photos and videos are downloaded and inserted into the slide presentation.

The cross: Two lines must be placed on the center of the slide, forming a cross (Figure 3.2). The full-face photo with the teeth apart should be positioned behind the cross.

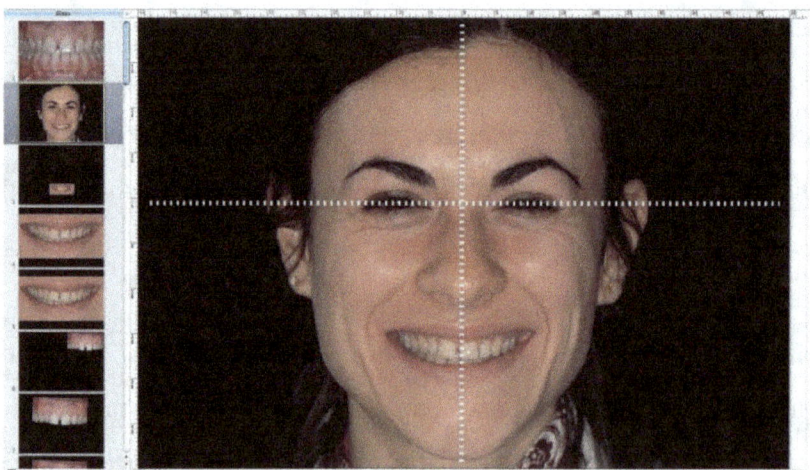

Figure 3.1: The DSD protocol can be utilized on the Keynote software or MS PowerPoint using the Digital Face Bow procedure. The face photo is placed on the slide to start the DSD sequence and is adjusted behind the two white dotted lines (the cross), determining visually the ideal facial midline and horizontal reference.

Digital facebow: Relating the full-face smile image to the horizontal reference line is the most important step in the smile design process. The interpupillary line should be the first reference to establish the horizontal plane, but it should not be the only one. It is also necessary to analyze the face as a whole and then determine the best horizontal reference that creates harmony. After determining the horizontal reference line, it is time to outline the facial midline according to facial features like the glabella, nose, and chin (Figure 3.1)

Smile analysis: Dragging the horizontal line over the mouth will allow an initial evaluation of the relation between the facial lines and the smile. It is possible to evaluate midline and occlusal plane shifting and/or canting (Figure 3.2).

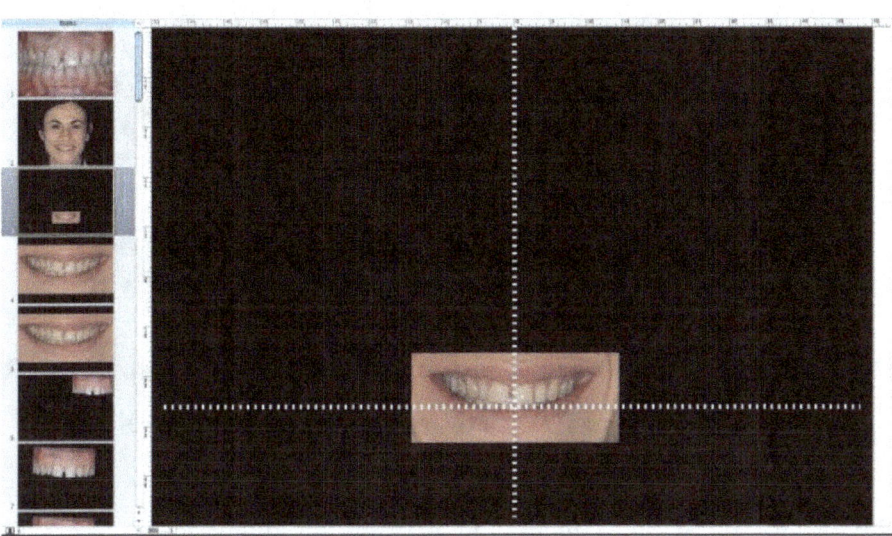

Figure 3.2: The horizontal line is moved to the mouth area and the face photo is cropped showing only the overall smile.

Smile Simulation: Simulations can be done to fix incisal edge position, canting, shifting, tooth proportion, and soft tissue architecture (Figure 3.3).

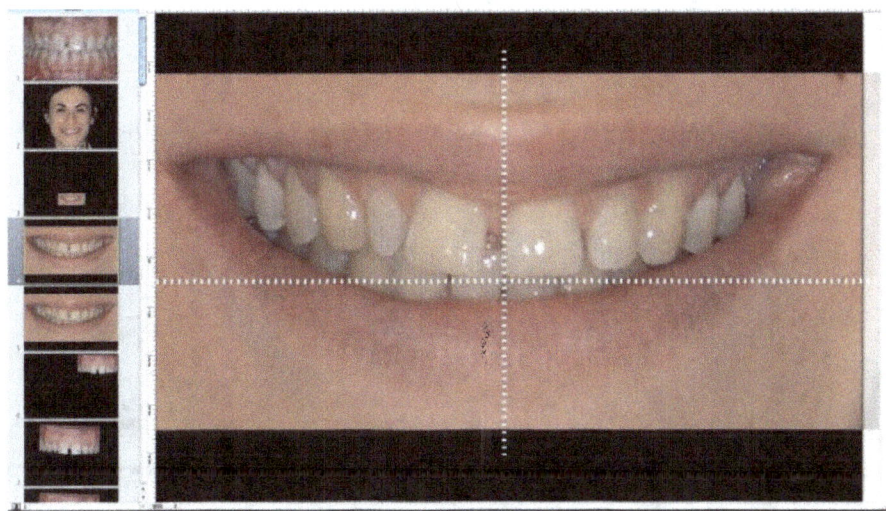

Figure 3.3: The smile and cross are enlarged to fill the whole slide.

Transference from the face to intraoral: In order to analyze the intraoral photo in accordance with the facial references one needs to transfer the cross to the retracted photo using three transferring lines drawn over the smiling photo (Figure 3.4):

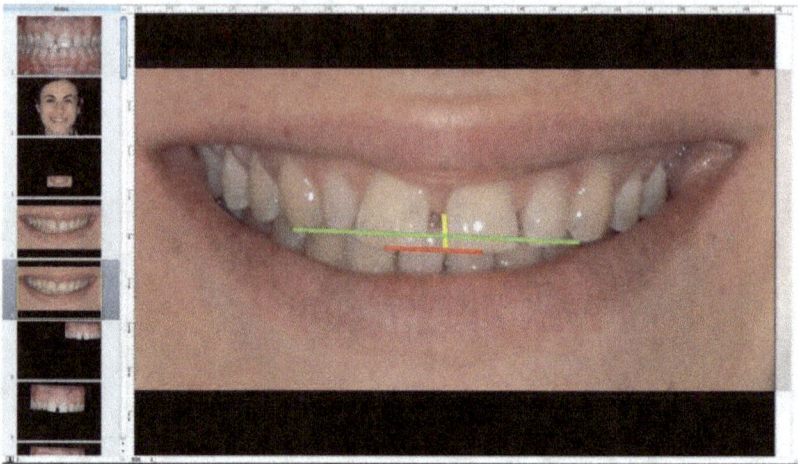

Figure 3.4: Three transferring lines are created. Green line: cuspid tips. Red line: incisal edge of the central. Yellow line: mesial of the central incisor.

Line 1: from the cusp tip of one canine to the tip of the contralateral canine.

Line 2: from the middle of the incisal edge of one central to the middle of the incisal edge of the other central.

Line 3: over the dental midline, from the tip of the papilla to the incisal embrasure. Thus, four features on the photo should be calibrated: size, canting, incisal edge position, and midline position. Line 1 guides the two first aspects (size and canting); line 2 guides the incisal edge position, and line 3 guides the midline position (Figure 3.5).

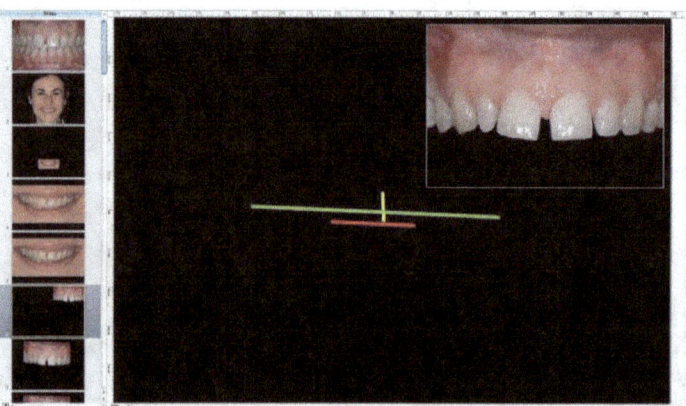

Figure 3.5: The three lines will be used to calibrate the intraoral photo to the facial cross.

6. **Measuring tooth proportion**: Measuring the width/length proportion of the central by placing a rectangle over the edges of the central (Figure 3.6) is an effective way to start understanding what needs to be performed when it comes to redesigning a smile. The other analysis that should be performed is to compare the actual proportion of the patient's central in relation to ideal proportions according to literature 2–9 (Figure 3.7).

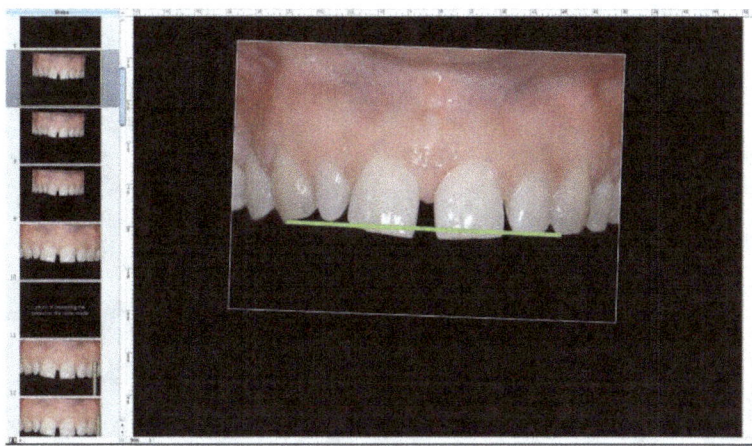

Figure 3.6: The first step to calibrate the intraoral photo is to adjust the size and inclination of the photo so that the cusp tips are touching the ends of the green line, exactly as performed on the facial photo.

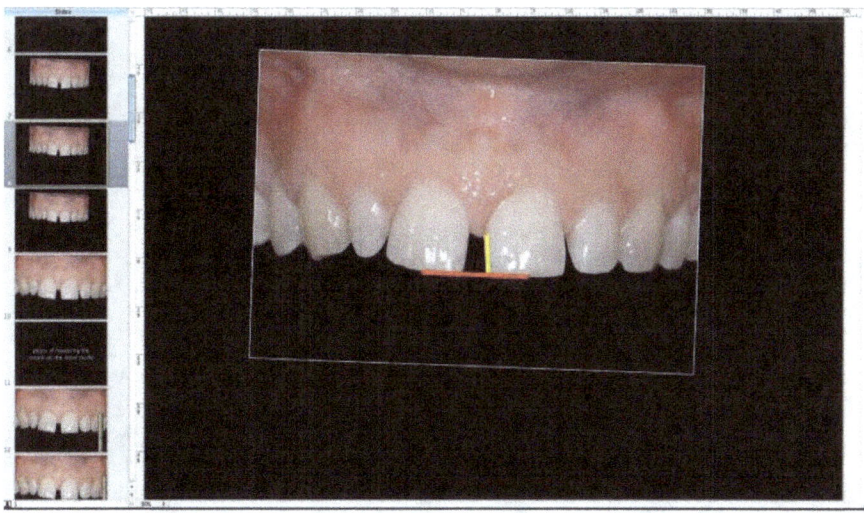

Figure 3.7: Step 2 is to move the photo so that the incisal edges and midline are touching the lines, exactly as performed on the face photo.

7. **Tooth outline**: From this point on, all the drawings may be customized, depending on the case, what you want to visualize, and what you want to communicate with the team, technician, and patient. One can draw the teeth outlines over the photo or copy and paste a pre-made outline from a personal library. The selection of the shape of the teeth will depend on other factors such as the morpho-psychological interview, the patient's desires, facial features, and esthetic expectations. 10, 11 (Figures 3.9 and 3.10).

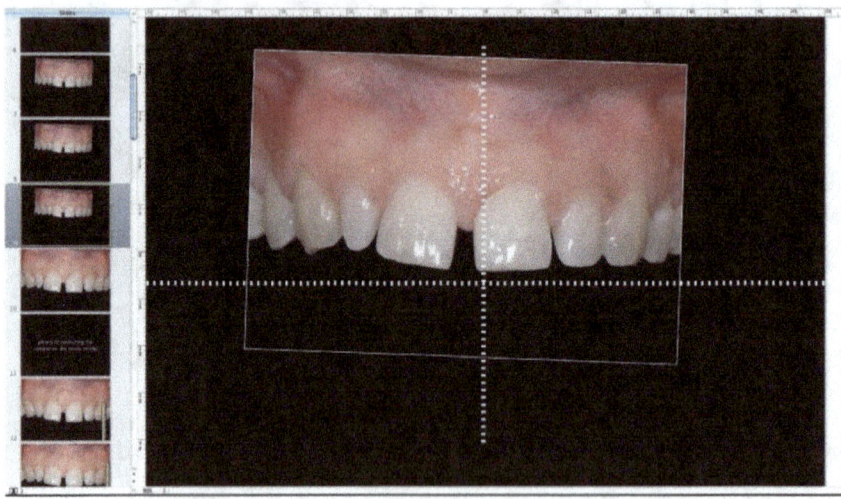

Figure 3.9: The dotted white lines are reintroduced into the slide and now the intraoral photo is calibrated with the facial cross.

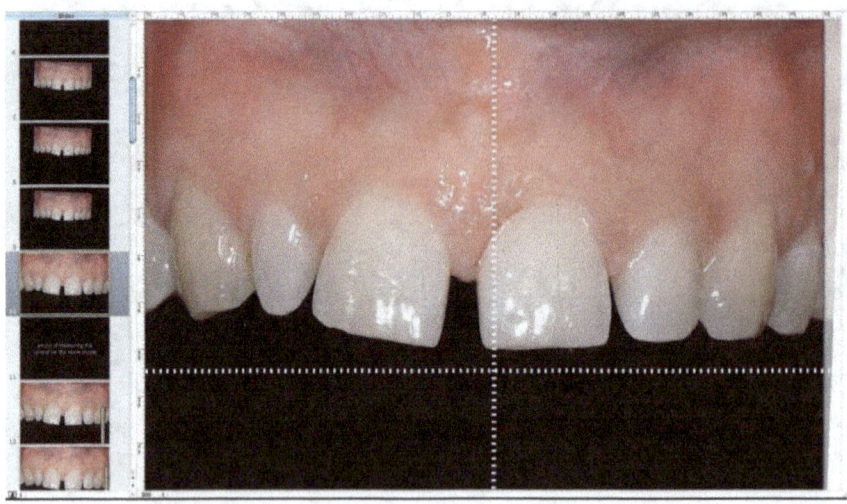

Figure 3.10: The lines and photo are positioned and stretched to fill in the whole slide, improving the visualization of the relationship between teeth, soft tissues, and the facial cross.

8. **White and pink esthetic evaluation**: After having all the lines and drawings performed according to the facial lines and the smile line, one can have a clear understanding of all the esthetic issues involving the upper arch such as tooth proportion, interdental relationship, the relationship between the teeth and the smile line, discrepancy between facial and dental midline, midline and occlusal plane canting, soft tissue disharmony, the relationship between soft tissue and teeth, papillae heights, gingival margin levels, incisal edge design, tooth axis, and so on (Figure 3.11).

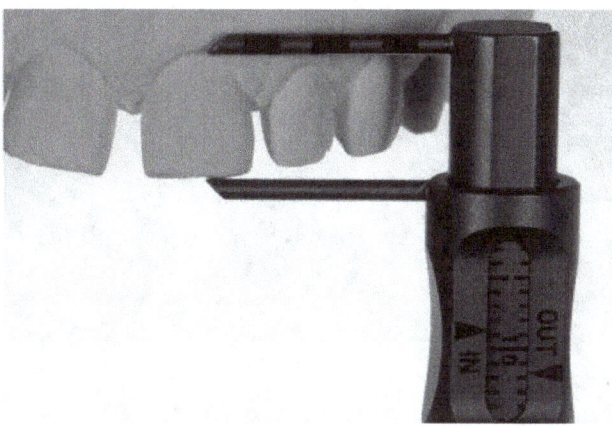

Figure 3.11: With a caliper measure the real length of the central incisor on the stone model (8mm). This measurement will be used to calibrate the Digital Ruler

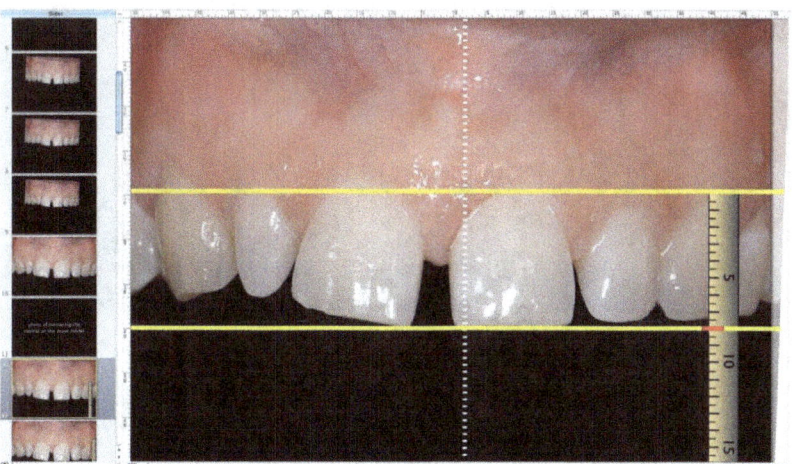

Figure 3.12: Using the computer again, the Digital Ruler is dragged onto the slide and calibrated according to the 8mm measurement obtained. The zero on the ruler is placed on one of the yellow horizontal lines and then the ruler is stretched or reduced until the #8 reaches the other yellow line.

9. **Digital Ruler calibration over the intraoral photo**: After all the lines are placed and drawings made, one can proceed with the calibration of the Digital Ruler over the intraoral photo by measuring the real length of one central incisor on the model (Figure 3.12) and transferring this measure to the computer (Figure 3.13). Once the Digital Ruler is calibrated one can start making any kind of measurements over the anterior area of the image (Figure 3.14).

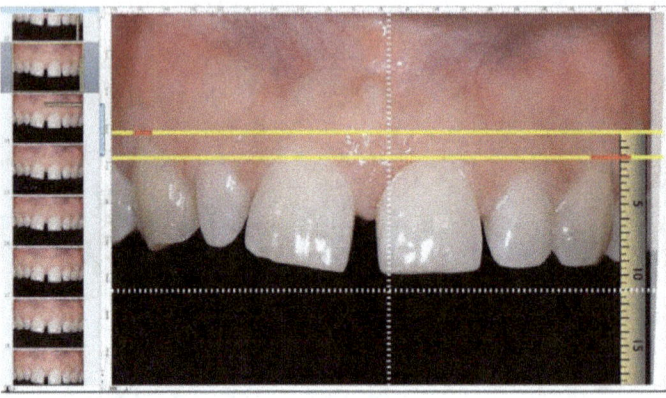

Figure 3.13: After calibration, measurements can be performed on top of the photo on the anterior area. For example, the discrepancy between the heights of the cervical of the cuspids is 1.7mm.

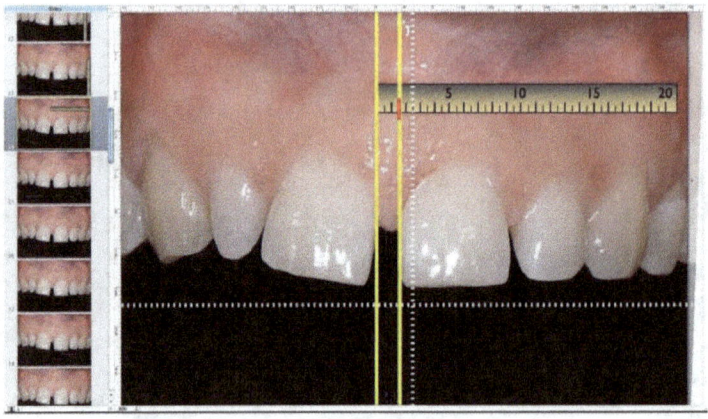

Figure 3.14: Measure the diastema, 1.5mm.

10. **Transferring the cross from digital to the model**: The first step is to digitally move the horizontal line over the intraoral photo and place it above the gingival margin of the six anterior teeth. With the Digital Ruler the distance is measured between the horizontal line and the gingival margin of each tooth and these sizes are written down on the slide (Figure 3.15). These measurements are transferred to the model with the aid of a caliper, marking on

the model with a pencil the same exact distances above the gingival margins that are shown on the computer and connecting the dots that create a horizontal line above the teeth. The next step is to transfer the vertical midline, perpendicular to the horizontal line. One should measure the distance between the dental midline and the facial midline at the incisal edge level on the computer and then transfer this mark to the model with the caliper (Figure 3.16). After drawing the cross on the model (Figure 3.17) it is possible to transfer the information digitally planned, such as crown lengthening, incisal edge reduction, root coverage, and so on. At this point all the information necessary for the technician to develop a precise and useful wax-up is on the slides and on the model, guiding him or her to best perform this procedure (Figure 3.18)

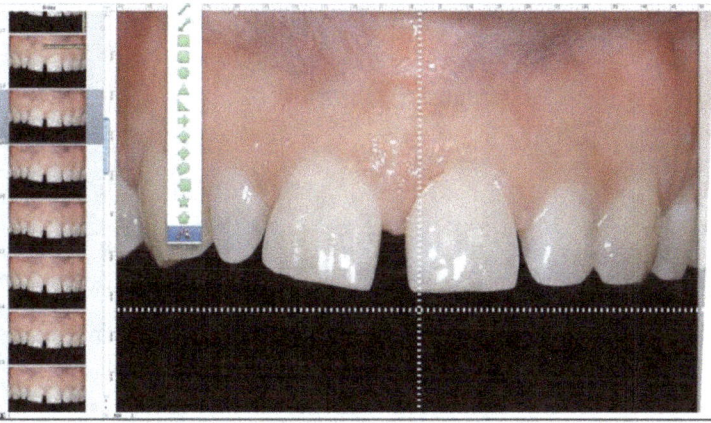

Figure 3.16: Make the digital drawings over the photo on the slide with the drawing tool.

The guided diagnostic wax-up is integrated with the patient's facial features and emotional needs.

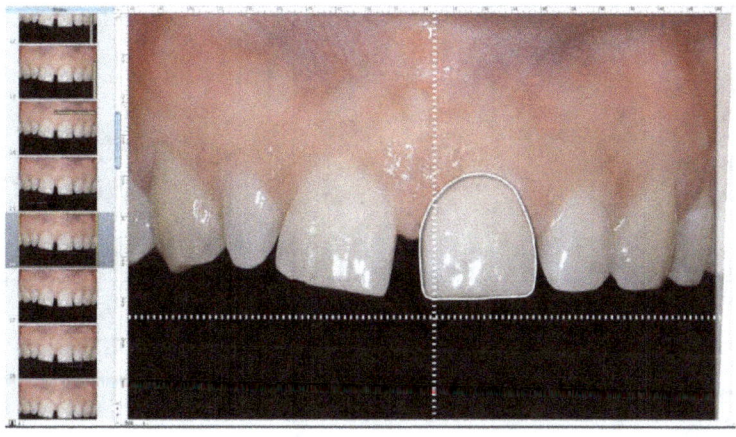

Figure 3.17: Draw the central incisor.

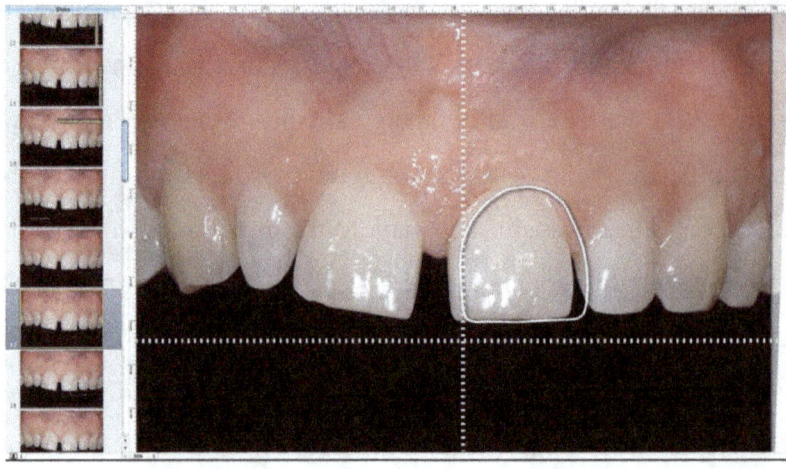

Figure 3.18: The Digital Mock-Up. Move the central distally to remove the distal diastema and to improve the match between the dental and facial midline.

The guided diagnostic wax-up is integrated with the patient's facial features and emotional needs.

The next important step is to evaluate the precision of the DSD and the wax-up by performing a "test drive" (Figure 3.19). It can be a mock-up or a provisional, depending on the case. After the patient's approval of the "test drive," one can plan and adapt all the following procedures to achieve the desired result. The tooth preparation should be minimally invasive allowing just enough clearance to create proper ceramic restorations (Figure 3.20).

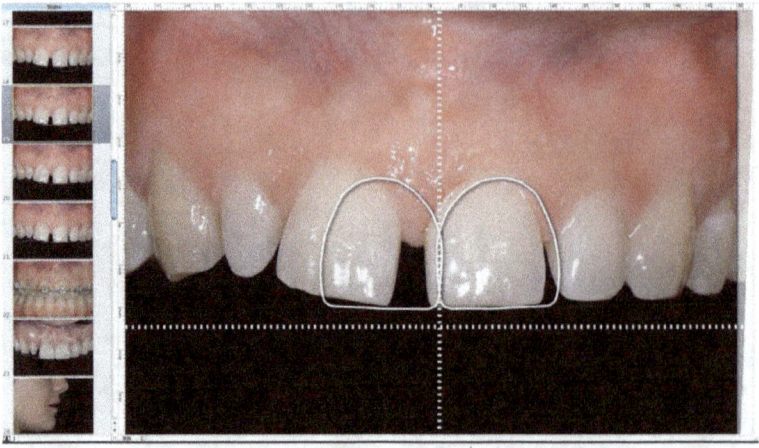

Figure 3.19: Flip the drawing and position it symmetrically to the other central. One can immediately visualize the difference between the actual and ideal position of the right central.

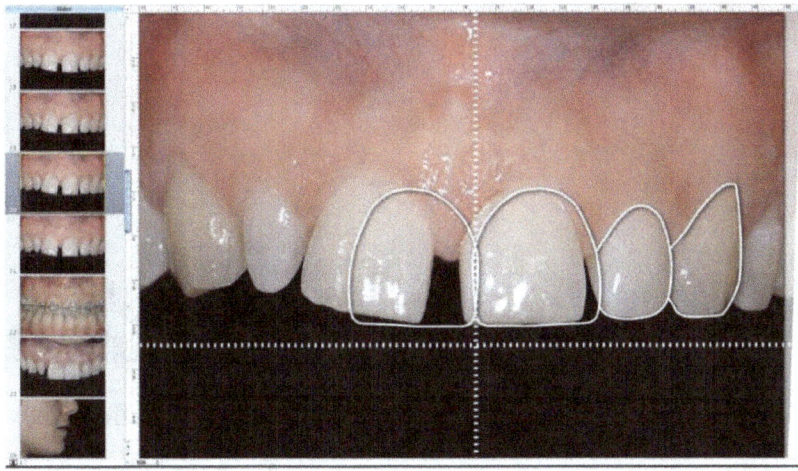

Figure 3.20: Draw the left lateral and cuspid to serve as a reference for the ideal position of the contralateral teeth.

The fabrication of the final restorations should be a controlled process with very few final adjustments (Figure 3.21), and the final result should be completely integrated, exceeding the patient's expectations (Figures 3.22 and 3.23).

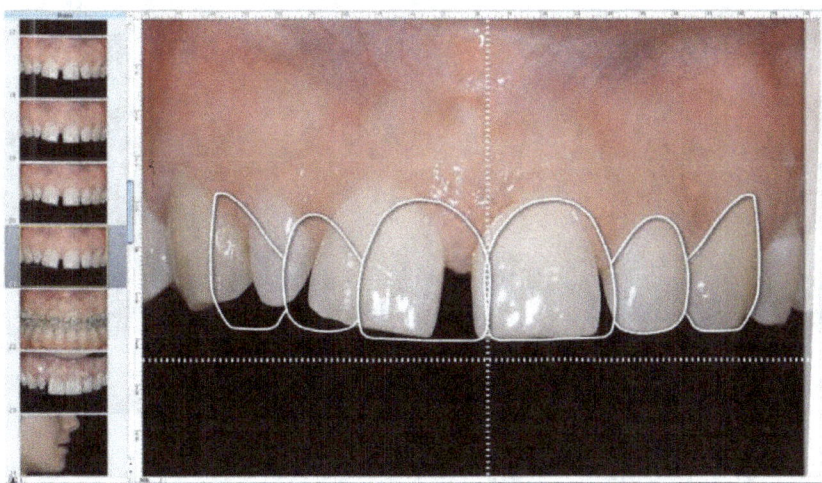

Figure 3.21: Flip and position the lateral and cuspid drawings symmetrically in order to visualize the discrepancy between the actual and ideal positions of the six anterior teeth. This can demonstrate to the orthodontist the movements required as well as show the patient the necessity of orthodontics to allow for minimally invasive preparations for veneers.

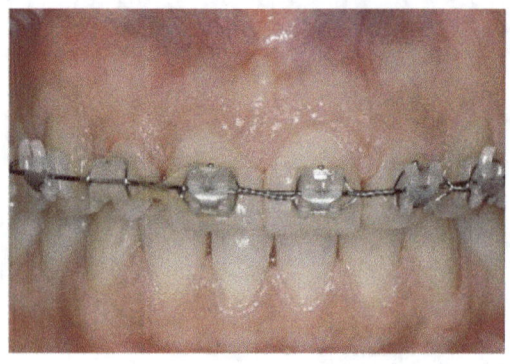

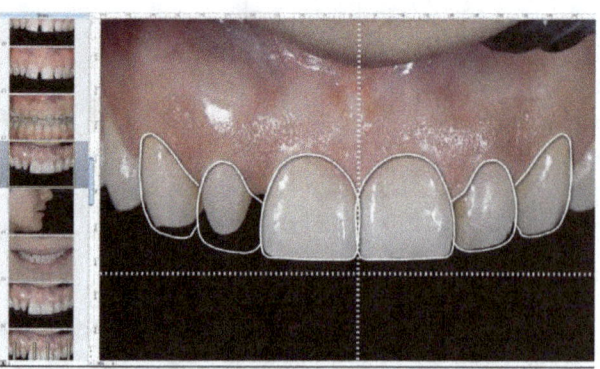

Figure 3.22: Situation after orthodontics.

Figure 3.23: The effectiveness of ortho treatment can be visualized by superimposing the digital planning drawings over the post-treatment photo.

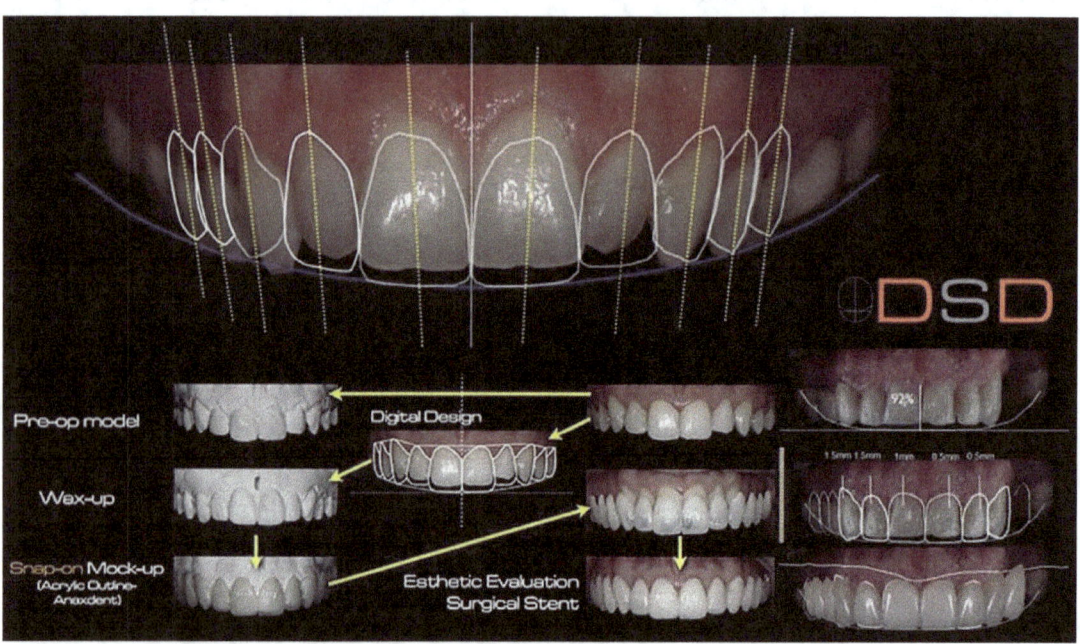

Figure 3.24: Digital planning for the restorative procedures. Analyzing the relation between the length of the anterior. The first guess is about how much one can lengthen the anterior.

REFERENCES

1. **Coachman C, Van Dooren E, Gürel G, et al.** Smile design: from digital treatment planning to clinical reality. In: Cohen M, ed. Interdisciplinary Treatment Planning. Vol. II: Comprehensive Case Studies. Hanover Park, IL: Quintessence; 2011.
2. **Rufenacht CR.** Fundamentals of Esthetics. Carol Stream, IL: Quintessence; 1990.
3. Dawson PE. Functional Occlusion: From TMJ to Smile Design. St Louis, MO: Mosby; 2007.
4. **Spear FM.** The maxillary central incisor edge: a key to esthetic and functional treatment planning. Compend Contin Educ Dent 1999;20(6):512–516.
5. **Goldstein RE.** Esthetics in Dentistry: Principles, Communication, Treatment Methods. Ontario, ON: B. C. Decker; 1998.
6. **Chiche GJ, Pinault A.** Esthetics of Anterior Fixed Prosthodontics. Hanover Park, IL: Quintessence; 1996.
7. **Magne P, Belser U.** Bonded Porcelain Restorations in the Anterior Dentition: A Biomimetic Approach. Carol Stream, IL: Quintessence; 2002.
8. **Fradeani M.** Esthetic Rehabilitation in Fixed Prosthodontics: Esthetic Analysis: A Systematic Approach to Prosthetic Treatment. Carol Stream, IL: Quintessence; 2004.
9. **Gürel G.** The Science and Art of Porcelain Laminate Veneers. Berlin: Quintessence; 2003.
10. **Paolucci B.** Visagism and dentistry. In: Hallawell P, ed. Integrated Visagism: Identity, Style, and Beauty. São Paulo: Senac; 2009:243–250.
11. **Paolucci B, Gürel G, Coachman C, et al.** Visagism: the Art of Smile Design Customization. São Paulo: VM Cultural; 2011.

CHAPTER-4

DENTAL PHOTOGRAPHY

Photography has always been an integral part of dentistry. The journey goes back to the time when film photography was used only for documentation and referral purposes which have now evolved into digital photography.

Digital photography has now penetrated into all the segments of science, medicine, industry, fashion designing, communication, and arts, and it would be difficult to imagine any form of our existence without photography. It has influenced the conscience of people so much that the saying "an image is worth a thousand words" is accepted as an undeniable fact.

of dentistry and photography began in 1840 when the first dental school was opened with the world's first photographic gallery and was operated by a dentist turned photographer. Since then, photography and dentistry have been partners as photography became an integral part of a patient's record and treatment plan.[1]

Photography provides the operator the ability to record patient data, events, and document scientific discoveries in a unique way. **Alexander Wolcott** (1804–1844) played a key role in the history of photography. He obtained the patent for his invention of the camera in 1840 and developed a system for photographic studio lighting. Soon after 1 month, he made history by opening the first commercial photographic studio.[1] In 1848, **Dr. R. Thompson and W. Elde** of Columbus, Ohio, marked the first time use of before and after photographs of a dental procedure, and an article was published creating a new frontier in diagnosis and treatment planning.

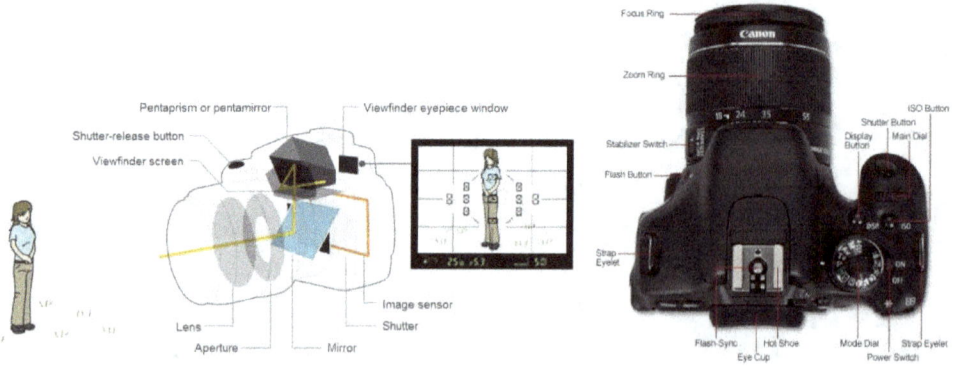

FIGURE 4.1: PARTS OF A DSLR CAMERA

The History

More recently, the dental profession has started to use clinical photography as part of diagnostic and treatment planning processes. Its value in documenting cases, presenting information, and educating patients has increased to the point that it has become integral to diagnosis and treatment planning decisions to be taken as required for the procedures.[1]

Digital photography arrived in the mid-1990 with digital cameras available at the marketplaces. Although its resolution was low, it had already started to create ripples of interest among purists and enthusiasts. Within 10 years or so, digital photography has completely displaced film photography in science and medicine. The new software has come which allows things to be measured, changed, shared, and integrated into new communication tools with just a click of a mouse. The images also can now be animated, used in reports, and published on websites. These applications are unparalleled in film technologies.[2]

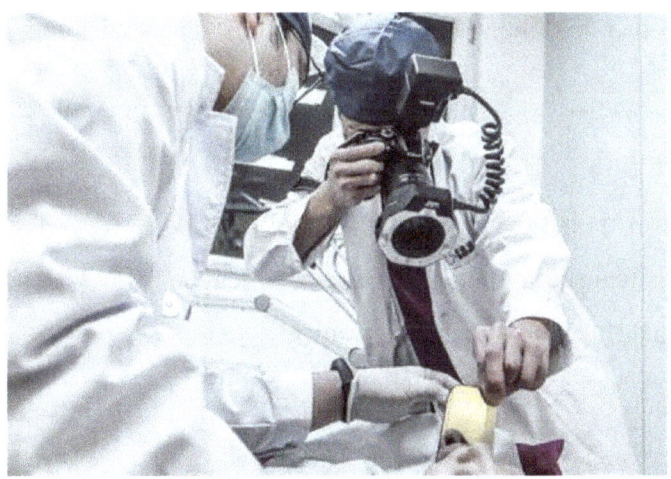

FIGURE 4.2: DIGITAL DENTAL PHOTOGRAPHY

REASONS WHY TO USE DIGITAL DENTAL PHOTOGRAPHY

With the advent of digital technologies, imaging has now become easier and more readily accessible. Still, few are reluctant to implement them in their daily practices for reasons such as lack of knowledge of photography equipment and technique, interruption in workflow, and cost factors. However, as new technologies are continuously emerging, the equipment cost is declining as well, thus every practitioner can implement photography into his or her practice with minimal interruptions in their patient workflow. The following are the reasons why to use digital dental photography in everyday dental practice:

Diagnosis and treatment planning.

There are 34 views required for all clinical case examinations. Of the 34 views, 17 should be taken before treatment and 17 after treatment. Additional views are required for the technical documentation. The images should be captured in either manual or TTL mode. All intraoral images should be captured using high F-stops to maximize the depth of field.[2,3] Intraoral and extraoral photographs provide a static, in-depth look at the patient's dentition and profile, which can be easily reviewed and compared with the other patient records[2]

Enhanced patient education and communication

Till now, there were audio and visual aids such as videos, models, and brochures, for patient education purposes, but none of these modalities thoroughly covered the information. Utilizing a tablet display and presentation software, tailored presentations on dental procedures could be created with photographed cases. These detailed pictures showing anatomy, surgical steps, materials, and completed cases can help in educating the patients on diagnosis and proposed treatment and thereby improving their understanding and case acceptance.[2,3]

Legal Documentation

Digital photographs in their raw format (nonedited) can be used as legal document proof. This can help a mistreated patient or defend a colleague who has provided appropriate treatment or can be helpful in malpractice lawsuits.[2,3]

Insurance verification

Periodontal charting, radiographs, or a narrative is required by insurance companies before the disbursement of benefits to the consumer. Therefore, a digital photograph can be used to support a narrative.[2,3]

Specialist consultation

Charted radiographs and written reports were the only means to present our patients to other doctors. Now, with photographs, an entirely new dimension has been introduced. A complete case history with high-resolution photographs may be sufficient enough for an over-the-phone consultation with a specialist. Similarly, photographs from referring dentists of mutual patients and their recent accomplishments could be transferred or received so that the operator may assess the condition without being physically present in the office.[2,3]

Laboratory communication

A shade guide is often required to convey information on the tooth or gingival character, shade, or color. This procedure is mostly accompanied by demerits like falling short in describing the complexity of depth and shadowing a tooth exhibits. Hence, here, a color-corrected photograph can provide the much-needed information to create a final restoration with a more accurate hue, value, and chroma.[2,3]

Professional advertising and marketing

Before and after photos are powerful aids to motivate the patients for accepting the treatment plan or for showcasing any particular skill.[2,3]

Professional instruction

Only texts and bullets are often inadequate in describing dental concepts or specific surgical procedures.

A photo is worth more than a thousand words and sparks more interest and discussion than a written matter under discussion.[2,3]

Self-education/improvement

As professionals, we continuously learn throughout our careers. Courses and other forms of continuing education are important educational vehicles. Digital photography on such occasions is a blessing in disguise.[2,3]

Treatment philosophy and work ethic

Taking efforts and time to clean surgical sites for photographs requires patience and painstaking attention to detail. This attitude propels us to execute our work at high levels of accuracy. Hence, preparing the patient for photographs helps improve our skills.[2,3]

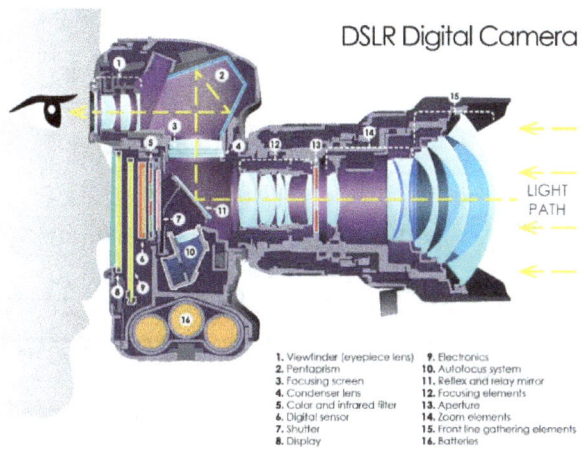

Basic armamentarium

The following is the list of basic instruments required for digital dental photography:

1. Digital camera[7]

   FIGURE 4.3 IMAGE DEPICTING PARTS OF A DIGITAL CAMERA

   - Compact point-and-shoot cameras or
   - Digital single-lens reflex

     More the pixels, the greater would be the detail of the image. In digital dental photography, a minimum of 10 Mega Pixels is required.

   - Intraoral cameras

2. Camera accessories:

   - Lens:

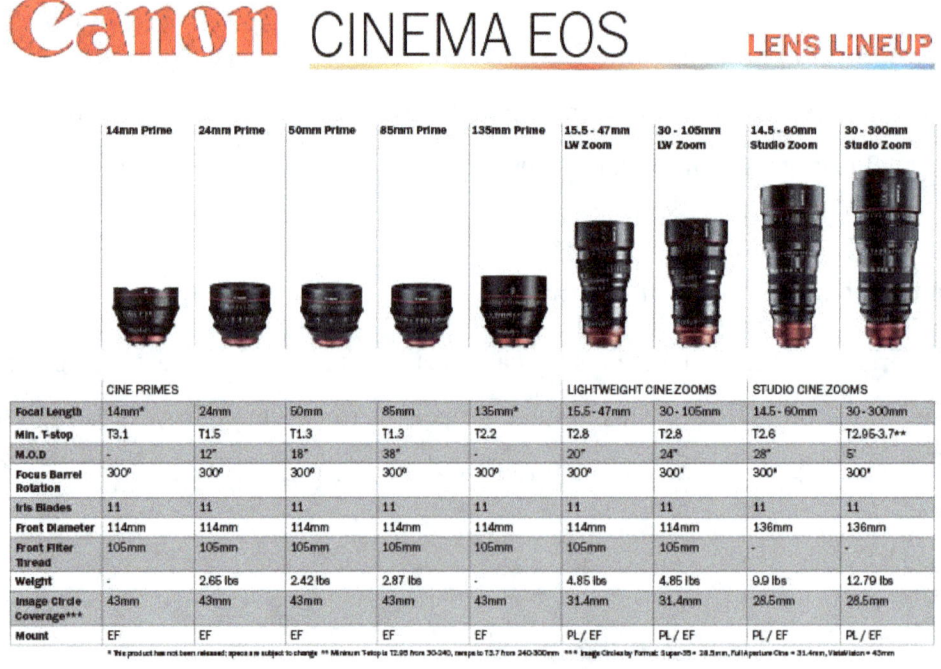

Figure 4.4: Various sizes of macro lenses

The macro-lens of the fixed focal length of 85–105 mm. There are different types of lenses available and each one is for different uses. The lens that mostly concerns us for documentation and record purposes is mainly micro-lenses. These lens systems allow a sharper focus in the close-up pictures as they have a larger diaphragm and we get a higher magnification than with other armature lenses. In medical and technical documentation, the objects and the images are dealt with in close ranges. Using a macro lens will help the user to focus better and obtain sharper images.[4,5] These macro lenses are further distinguished from one another by the focal length, which varies from one lens to another. Focal lengths are normally 16 mm, 28 mm, 35 mm, 50 mm, 85 mm, 100 mm, 135 mm, 200 mm, 300 mm, 400 mm, etc. The lenses that are of interest for medical and technician offices are mainly those with a focal length of about 100 mm approximately.[4,5]

These lenses have mechanisms that are defined by the term "Diaphragm;" it consists of sheets that let more or less light in it, similar to the function of the iris in the human eye. With poor light, the diaphragm expands to let lighter pass through; on the other hand, if there is plenty of light, the diaphragm closes to the minimum to be able to see without being blinded. The aperture size or diaphragm width directly affects the sharpness of the image. As smaller the diaphragm size, the sharper would be the image.[6]

Hence, with true macro lenses, the operator can take advantage of the depth of field and obtain sharper and more focused images at their original magnification.

- o Light and electronic flash systems

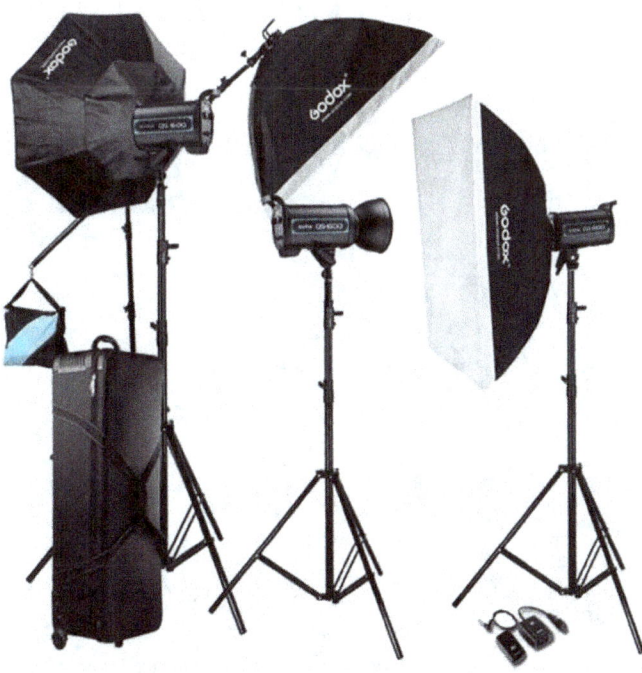

FIGURE 4.5: FLASH SYSTEM SETUP

a) Ring flash

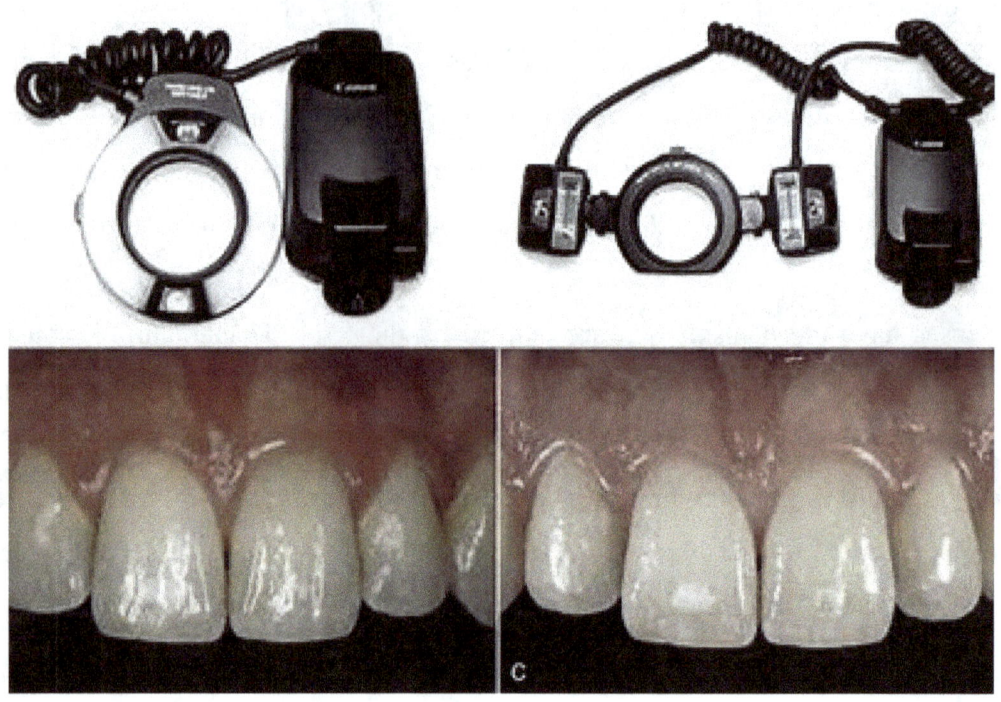

FIGURE 4.6: IMAGE DEPICTING THE DIFFERENCE OF ILLUMINATION USING DIFFERENT RING FLASH SYSTEM

b) Point flash

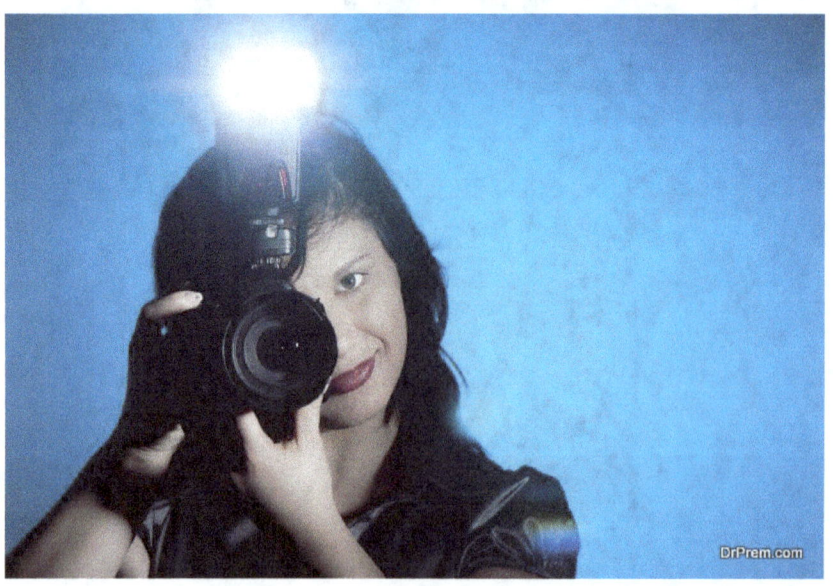

FIGURE 4.6: POINT FLASH

c) Twin flash

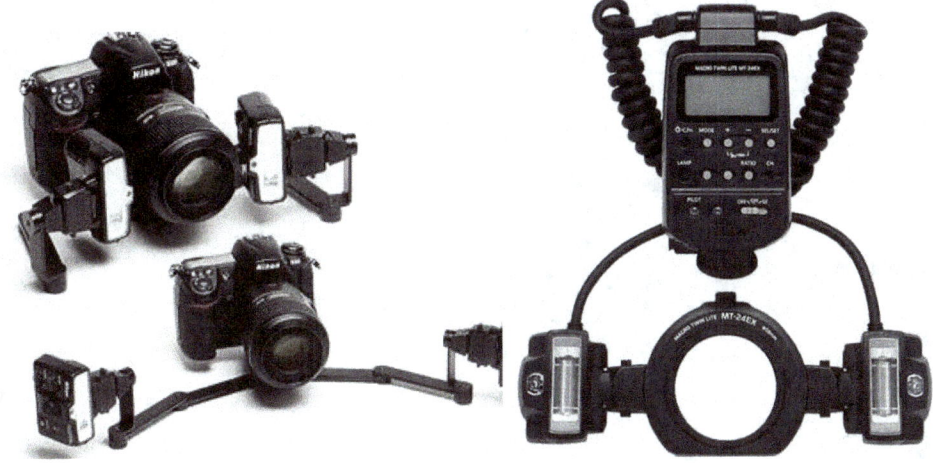

FIGURE 4.7 TWIN FLASH SYSTEMS USED IN DENTAL PHOTOGRAPHY

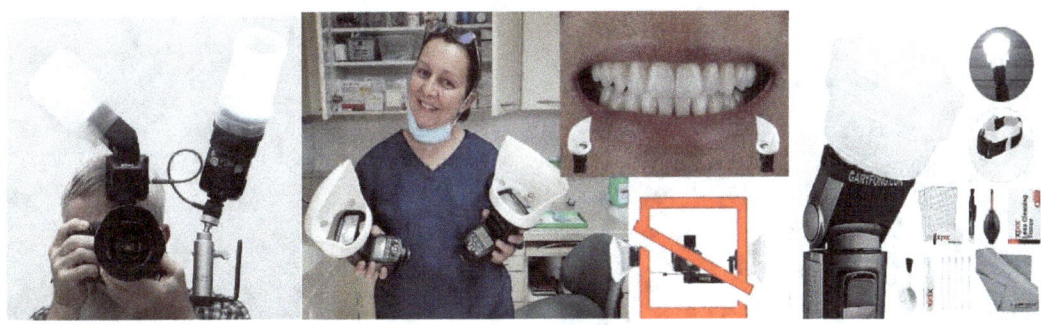

FIGURE 4.8: FLASH DIFFUSERS/ FILTERS

- o Memory card: for storage of data[7]

- o Filter: It serves the dual purpose of lens protection and if required changing the lighting conditions[7]

- o Batteries: An extra battery pack with a quick charger ensure that we never run out of battery during shoot[7]

- o Camera bags: These are useful to protect the camera and be able to carry our lens, camera, and other accessories in an organized fashion[7]

3. Clinical dentistry photographic accessories
    - o Cheek retractors

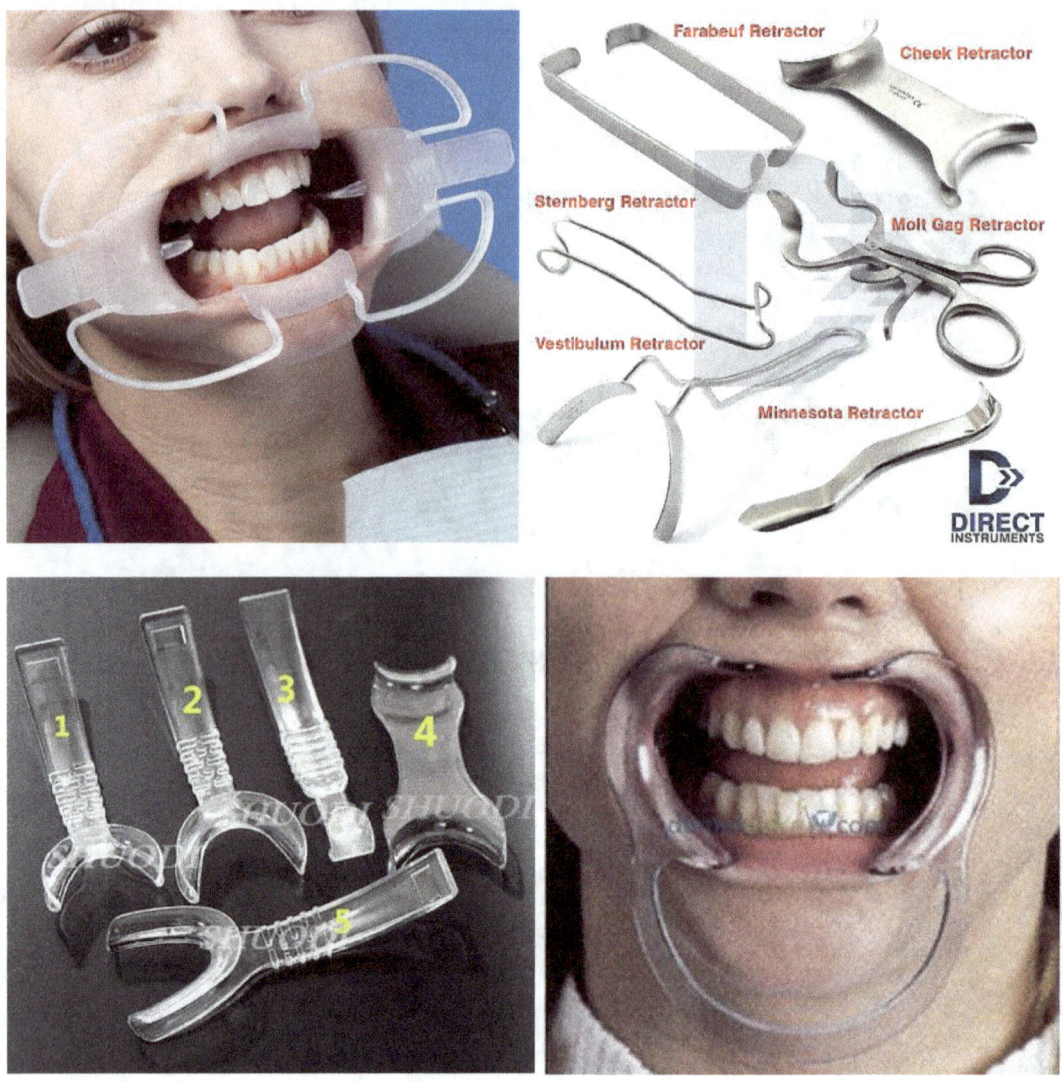

FIGURE 4.9 VARIOUS TYPES OF CHEEK RETRACTORS

a) Columbia wire lip retractor: This combines buccal mirror and cheek retractors[7]

b) The Martin metal retractors[7]

c) Intraoral mirrors: Like long-handled front-silvered rhodium-coated glass mirrors.[7]

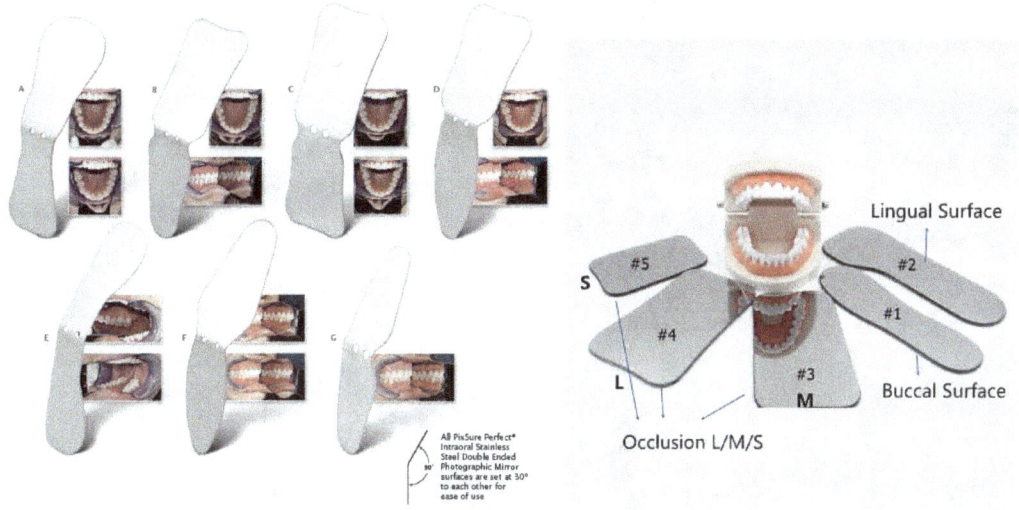

FIGURE 4.10: INRA-ORAL MIRRORS

- Black background/contrasters[7]

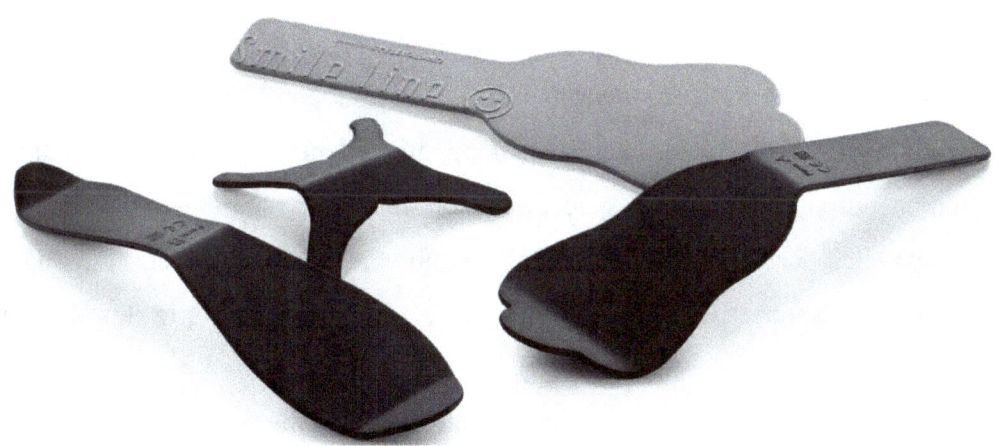

FIGURE 4.11: DENTAL PHOTOGRAPHY CONTRASTERS

4. Other accessories equipment for intraoral photography[7]:

   o Plastic or glass spatula

   o Disposable plastic spoons

   o Dental mirrors

   o Gauze strips

   o Air syringes or aspirators.

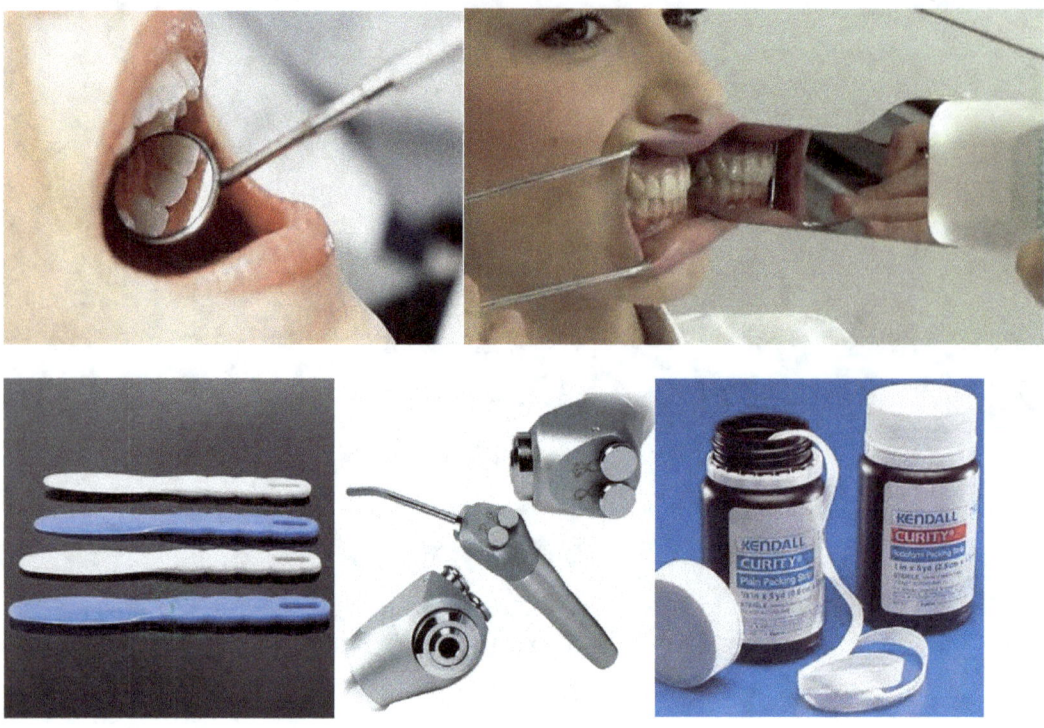

FIGURE 4.12: INTRA-ORAL ACCESSORIES USED IN DENTAL PHOTOGRAPHY

Dental photography has its own impact. Through digital photography, the operator can communicate with the patient as well as among other dentists for referral or treatment documentation purpose. Technical aspects such as smile line, smile width, facial profile, emergence profile, occlusal plane, gingival anatomy, compensatory curves, and shade matching can be better visualized through perfect intraoral and profile photographs.

It also brings laboratory cases closer to the visualization of the actual patient. With more information at disposal, operators and technicians can deliver better skills to a greater precision and achieve the patient's desired restorative outcome with lifelike results.

REFERENCES

1. **Galante DL.** History and current use of clinical photography in orthodontics. J Calif Dent Assoc 2009; 37:173-4.
2. **Bengel W.** Mastering Digital Dental Photography. 1st ed. New Maiden, Surry (UK): Quintessence Publishers; 2006.
3. **Yoo A.** 10 reasons why dental photography should be an essential part of your practice. Dent Econ 2014; 104:1-7.
4. **Manjunath SG, Raju Raghavendra T, Setty SK, Jayalakshmi K.** Photography in clinical dentistry – A review. Int J Dent Clin 2011; 3:40-3.
5. **Chandni P, Anupam S, Nitin S, Shikha G.** An overview on dental photography. Int J Dent Health Sci 2016; 3:581-9.
6. **Alberto C.** Digital photography and documentation techniques in dentistry and dental technology. Zerodonto 2013; 1:1-103.
7. **Sreevatsan R, Philip K.** Digital photography in general and clinical dentistry- technical aspects and accessories. Int Dent J Stud Res 2015; 3:17-24.

CHAPTER-5
COMPOSITES

Composite resin restorations were first recommended as a potential substitute for silicate cement, acrylic resin, and metallic restorations after their introduction in the late 1960s. Unfortunately, a series of well-controlled clinical studies demonstrated that these first-version composite resins were still deficient for acceptable clinical purposes.[1-5] The clinical performance of the original formulations was disappointing.[6] Clinical applications resulted in shortcomings including inadequate wear resistance,[7-12] bulk fracture,[8-12] microleakage[7-8-13] (and consequential secondary caries[14-15]), marginal breakdown,[16] postoperative sensitivity,[16-17] improper interproximal contact and contour,[13] inadequate marginal adaptation,[17] color instability,[6-8] in-adequate polishability,[6] pulpal irritation,[10] and the potential need for endodontic therapy.[6]

Today, after 40 years of material science development and laboratory as well as clinical trials in human subjects, composite resins have been revalidated as all-purpose restorative materials.[18-22] Among the main reasons (esthetic and mechanical) for such an expanded clinical application of composite resins is their ability to incorporate into the demineralized tooth structure (i.e., enamel and dentin) through hybridization.

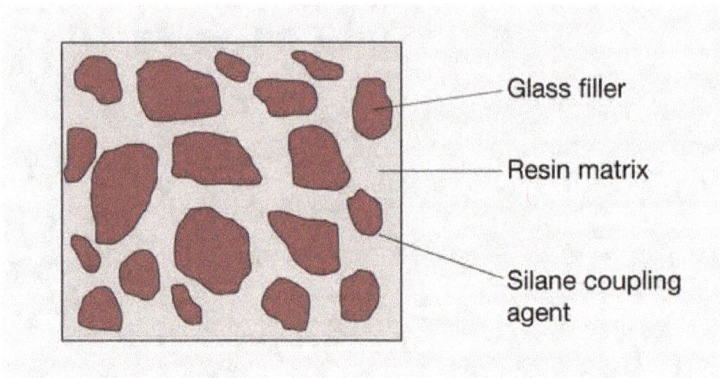

FIGURE 5.1: DENTAL COMPOSITE RESIN MATRIX

The term composite means a multiphase material formed from a combination of materials that differ in composition or form, remain bonded, and retain their identities and properties. Composites maintain an interface between components and act in concert to provide improved specific or synergistic characteristics not obtainable by any of the original components acting alone.[23]

Three phases comprise the infra-structure of composite resins: the organic phase (matrix), the dispersed phase (filler), and the interfacial phase (coupling agent).[24] Composite materials consist of a continuous polymeric or resin matrix in which an inorganic filler is dispersed.[22] The addition of fillers in dental composites significantly enhances their physical properties by increasing the strength and reinforcement of the matrix [25-29] while reducing the linear coefficient of thermal expansion.[30] Fillers include ground quartz, alumina silicate, pyrolytic silica, lithium aluminum silicates, borosilicate glass, and other types of glass, some of which contain oxides of heavy metals such as barium, strontium, zinc, aluminum, or zirconium (for radiopaque characteristics).[31-32] Produced by milling or grinding, precipitation, or through condensation, these fillers vary in particle size depending on the manufacturing process.

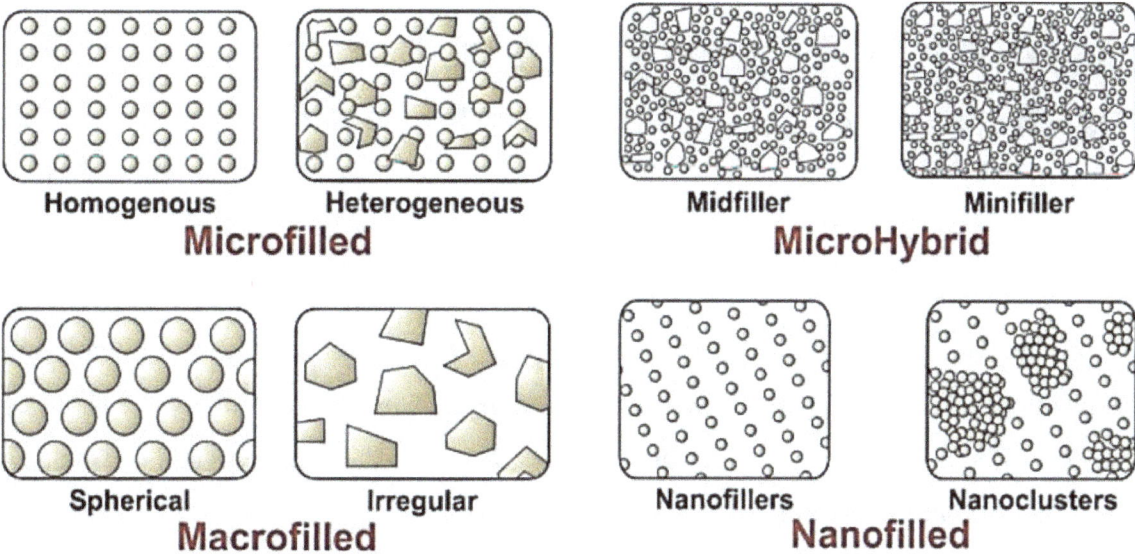

FIGURE 5.2: TYPES OF FILLER PARTICLES SIZE AND SHAPE IN DENTAL COMPOSITE RESINS

In composite resin technology, particle size and the number of particles represent crucial information in determining how best to utilize composite materials. Altering the filler component remains the most significant development in the evolution of composite resins.[33]

POLYMERIZATION SHRINKAGE

In a restorative procedure using composite resins, the polymerization reaction of the resin matrix phase can compromise dimensional stability.[34] This conversion of the monomer molecules into a polymer network is accompanied by a closer packing of the molecules, leading to bulk contraction.[35] Alternatively, when a curing material is bonded on all sides to rigid structures, bulk contraction cannot occur, and shrinkage must be compensated for by increased stress, flexure, or gap formation at the adhesive interface.[34]

The factors that influence polymerization shrinkage include the type of resin, the filler content of the composite, the elastic modulus of the material, curing characteristics,[36] water sorption, cavity configuration,[37], and the intensity of the light used to polymerize the composite.[38]

These undesirable effects can be managed and minimized with the following methods:[35]

- Application of cavity liners and bases that act as shock absorbers [39]

- Reduction of light intensity from curing units

- Incremental layering techniques of composite resins[40]

- Selection of low-shrinkage composite resin[41]

- Utilization of indirect composite resin restorations [38, 42, 43]

PLASTIC FILLING INSTRUMENTS

Composite and plastic filling instruments, also known as placement instruments, are designed for placing and contouring pliable restorative materials into cavity preparations and other dental procedures. These instruments generally have rounded ends that help in applying restoratives without damaging sensitive tissue.

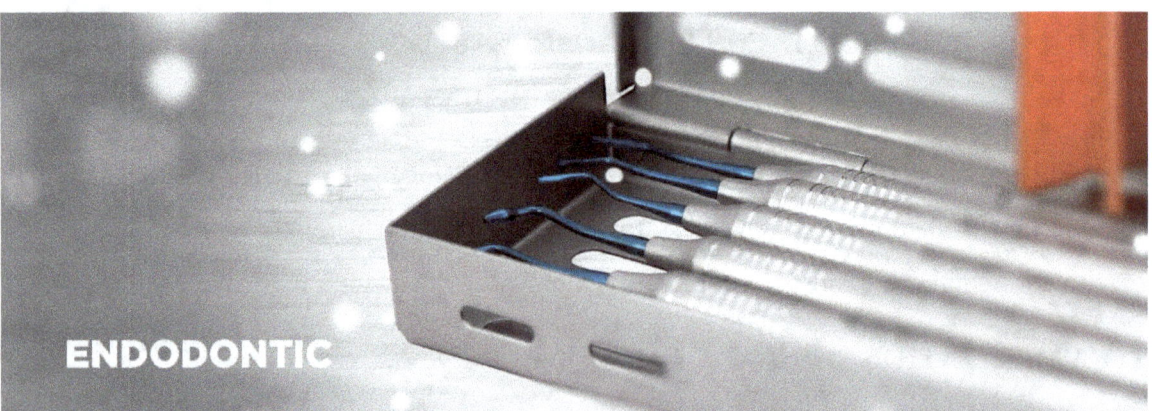

FIGURE5.3: PLASTIC FILLING INSTRUMENTS

Satin Steel XTS Composite Instruments – Posterior Composite Direct Fillings Medium/Large, Contact Forming, Double End

Satin Steel XTS are instruments for shaping, filing and placing composite or plastic material. All are made of highly polished stainless steel for nonstick applications. Various shapes and sizes to accommodate each procedure.

Area of Use: Posterior
Handle Material: Stainless Steel
Handle Shape: Round
Handle Type: XTS, Smooth Satin Steel
Manufacturer Name: Hu-Friedy Mfg Co. Inc.
Number of Ends: Double
Package Quantity: 1/Pkg

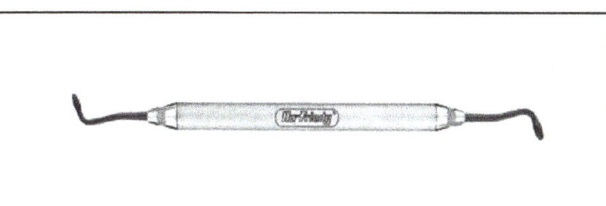

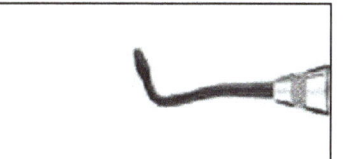

FIGURE 5.4: Satin Steel XTS
Tip Material: Stainless Steel
Tip Shape: Cone

Composite Instrument – Thin, Mini, Double – End # G3

Composite Instrument is used to contour composite and amalgam materials on large facial surfaces.

Area of Use: Facial
Design Number: G3
Manufacturer Name: PDT INC
Number of Ends: Double
Package Quantity: 1/Pkg

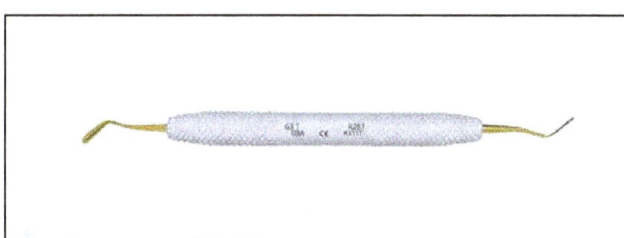

FIGURE5.5: Double – End # G3

COMPOSITES

Composite Instruments – # 3 Mini Goldstein, Anodized Aluminum, Double End

Goldstein Composite Instruments are lightweight, nonstick anodized aluminum instruments in a medium gray color. The #3 Mini is 1/3 smaller and thinner than Goldstein #3 and is used for reaching smaller, tighter areas such as lower incisors or deciduous teeth. This instrument is also excellent for packing gingival retraction cord around lower anteriors and tight sulcular areas.

Design Number: 3
Handle Material: Anodized Aluminum
Handle Shape: Round
Handle Type: Anodized Aluminum – Gray
Manufacturer Name: Hu-Friedy Mfg Co. Inc.

FIGURE 5.6: Double–End # G3

Number of Ends: Double
Package Quantity: 1/Pkg
Tip Material: Anodized Aluminum
Tip Type: Goldstein

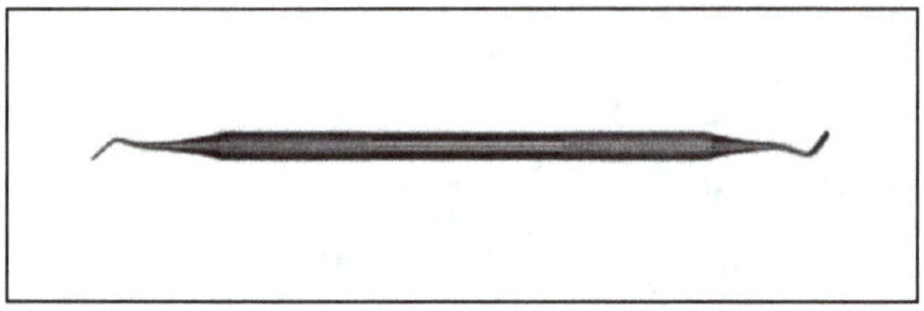

Cosmetic Contouring Instrument C – # 3 Goldfogel, Stainless Steel, Standard Handle, Double End

Goldfogel Cosmetic Contouring Instruments are used for placing and contouring composite and plastic dental material.

Design Number: 3
Handle Material: Stainless Steel
Handle Shape: Round
Handle Type: 10 Round
Manufacturer Name: Hu-Friedy Mfg Co. Inc.
Number of Ends: Double
Package Quantity: 1/Pkg
Tip Material: Stainless Steel

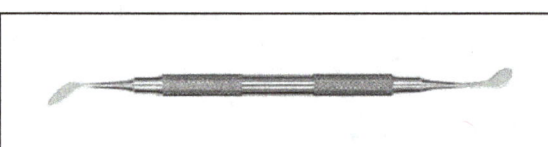

FIGURE 5.7: C – # 3 Goldfogel

Tip Shape: Paddle

Tip Type: Goldfogel

Composite/Plastic Filling Instruments with XP Technology™ – # 7 Paddle/Plugger, Standard Handle, Double End – 1/4″ Diameter

Composite Plastic Filling Instruments with XP Technology™ are made of titanium nitride, which is significantly harder than stainless steel, with a non-stick surface for packing, forming, and shaping composite materials.

Design Number: 7
Handle Diameter: 1/4″
Handle Material: Stainless Steel
Handle Type: Standard
Manufacturer Name: American Eagle Instruments
Number of Ends: Double
Package Quantity: 1/Pkg
Tip Diameter: 2 mm
Tip Material: Titanium Nitride
Tip Shape: Paddle, Plugger

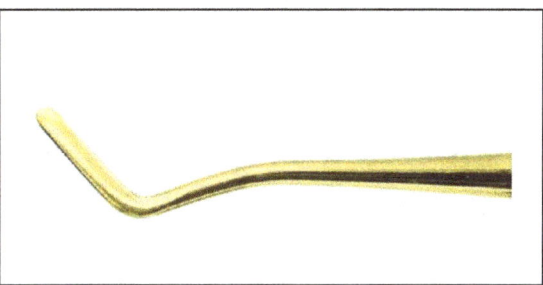

FIGURE 5.8: # 7 Paddle/Plugger

LM-Arte™ Solo Posterior Instrument, Double End

LM-Arte™ Solo Posterior Instrument is designed for esthetic restorations and direct veneering of the posterior teeth. The rounded and straight spatulas are especially suited for labial tooth surfaces.

Area of Use: Posterior
Handle Shape: Round
Manufacturer Name: PLANMECA INC
Number of Ends: Double
Package Quantity: 1/Pkg

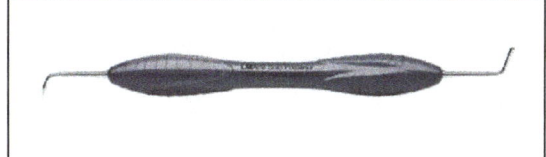

FIGURE 5.9: Solo Posterior Instrument

Goldstein Flexi-Thin Composite Instruments – 1, Double End – # 41 Round Handle

Goldstein Flexi-Thin Composite Instruments have thin, flexible, highly polished, non-stick, stainless-steel blades.

- #1 is a small universal style
- Rounded plugger tip
- Narrow paddle for initial placement and contouring of Class I, II and III restorations

Design Number: 1
Handle Material: Stainless Steel
Handle Shape: Round
Handle Type: 41 Round
Manufacturer Name: Hu-Friedy Mfg Co. Inc.

Number of Ends: Double
Package Quantity: 1/Pkg
Tip Material: Stainless Steel
Tip Shape: Paddle, Plugger
Tip Type: Goldstein

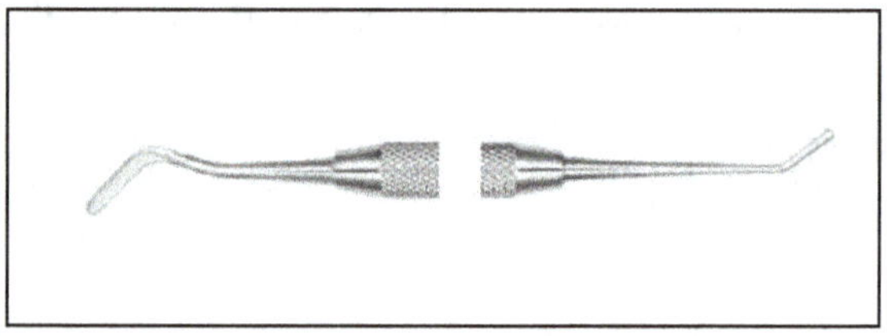

FIGURE 5.10 Flexi Thin Instrument

Plastic Filling Instruments – # 4 PFI, Standard Handle, Double End

Plastic Filling instruments are used to deliver restorative materials to the cavity preparation and contour the restorative materials.

Design Number: 4
Handle Type: Standard
Manufacturer Name: J&J Instruments Inc.
Number of Ends: Double
Package Quantity: 1/Pkg

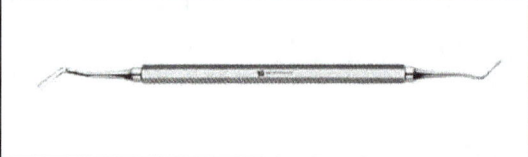

FIGURE 5.11: # 4 PFI

Microfil Composite Instruments, Double End – Carving, Blue

Almore Microfil Composite Instruments are lightweight and ideal for composite restoration development.

- Autoclavable
- Tips at the black end of instruments are replaceable
- Gold instrument is designed for use in the incisal area
- Green Instrument is designed for use in the gingival area
- Blue instrument is designed for carving

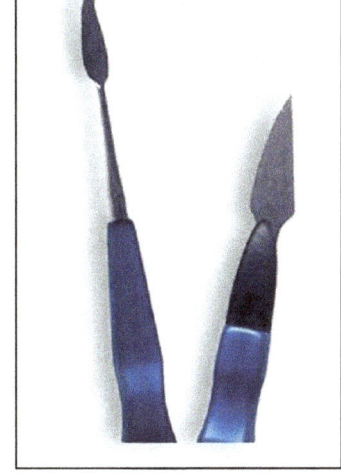

FIGURE 5.12: Almore Microfil

Manufacturer Name: Almore Mfg Company
Number of Ends: Double
Package Quantity: 1/Pkg
Tip Shape: Carver

Patterson® Composite and Plastic Filling Instruments – 6, Standard Handle, Double End – Anodized Aluminum

- Available in double-end anodized aluminum and stainless steel
- Anodized aluminum features nonstick surface that will not corrode or stain; lightweight handle improves tactile feel; black color makes these instruments easy to identify
- Both models are easy to clean
- Made in the USA

Design Number: 6
Handle Material: Anodized Aluminum
Handle Type: Standard
Manufacturer Name: Patterson Dental Supply
Number of Ends: Double
Package Quantity: 1/Pkg 44

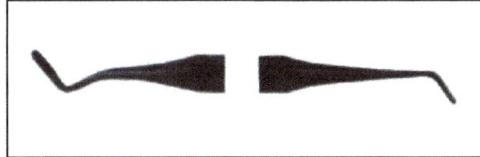

FIGURE 5.13: Patterson® Composite

OptraSculpt

OptraSculpt and OptraSculpt Pad are contouring instruments suitable for the non-stick shaping and contouring of surfaces45, 46, 47. They are especially designed to shape unpolymerized sculptable composites in direct restorative treatments and to contour and smoothen paste-like laboratory composites.

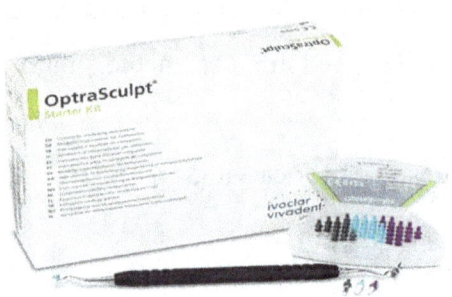

FIGURE 5.14: Optrasculpt

Easy adaptation

- Non-stick properties: reduce the stickiness of the composite versus the instrument45, 46, 47
- Compatibility: attachments are suitable for both instruments
- Working angles are adjusted to the anterior and posterior regions45, 46

Professional esthetics

- No marks left by the instrument on the restoration surface46, 47
- Reduction of air inclusions in the composite during application46, 47
- Homogeneous surface texture46, 47

High efficiency

- Efficient, easy contouring due to specially adjusted attachment shapes45, 46
- Reduced effort in finishing and polishing 46, 47

Efficient Esthetics

- OptraSculpt forms a part of the "Direct Restoratives" product category. The products of this category cover the procedure involved in the direct restoration of teeth – from preparation to restoration care. The products are optimally coordinated with each other and enable successful processing and application.

OptraSculpt Pad

- Foam pad attachments for non-stick, mark-free contouring[45, 46, 47]
- Two pad sizes for efficient contouring of direct veneers and large-surface class III and IV restorations
- Reference scale on the instrument handle for recording the axis alignment and the width of the anterior teeth[47]
- Optimum working angle for the anterior region[45, 46]

OptraSculpt Next Generation

- Three attachment shapes for the professional creation of sophisticated anatomical tooth structures: ball, pointed tip, chisel
- Optimum working angle for the posterior region[45, 46]
- Hygienic dispenser box for easy access to attachments

Cosmedent Composite Brushes

These applicator brushes for dental brushes applications come in 3 useful sizes. They are excellent for the application of opaques and tints, bonding adhesives, silanating agents, and cement removal prior to polymerization. Use the fine brush (#1) for fine detailing, and (#2) and (#3) brushes for the rest of your restorative dental needs.

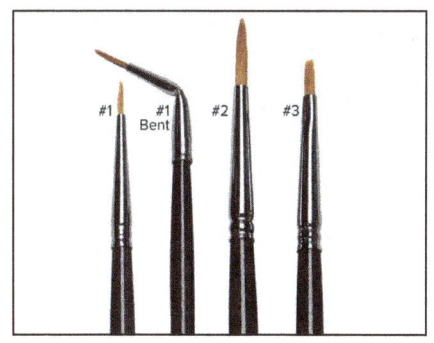

FIGURE 5.15: Cosmedent brushes

Advantages

- Composite silicone brushes facilitate a variety of dental resin applications
- Synthetic bristles make application easy

Indications for Use

- Use the fine #1 brush for fine detailing and application of tints and opaques
- Use the #2 and #3 brushes to apply bonding and silanating agents and for cement removal prior to polymerization.

Cleaning your composite brush

Chairside uses alcohol-dampened gauze to clean the composite brushes between materials.

In the lab/sterilization area:

- Soak the bristles in **Brush Cleaner** for a few minutes then wipe clean with gauze.
- Soak in cold sterilization fluid, follow the directions according to the manufacturer.
- Dry dental composite brushes and store them for the next patient.

CLASS I COMPOSITE RESTORATION

For oblique layering to the cavity wall: composite condenser (S-MTN, American Eagle Instruments).

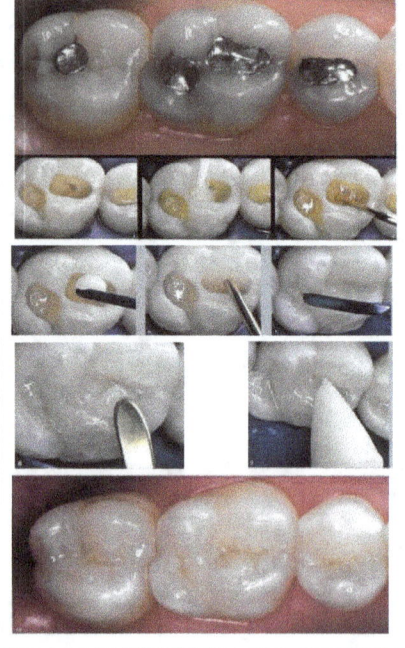

	Final pre-occlusal layer: long-bladed interproximal instrument
	A final enamel increment of incisal-shaded hybrid composite: a curved metal instrument (TINL-R, Brasseler USA)
	Polish was accomplished with an aluminum oxide-impregnated point (enhance finishing system, dentsply caulk)
	Final Restoration

CLASS II COMPOSITE RESTORATION

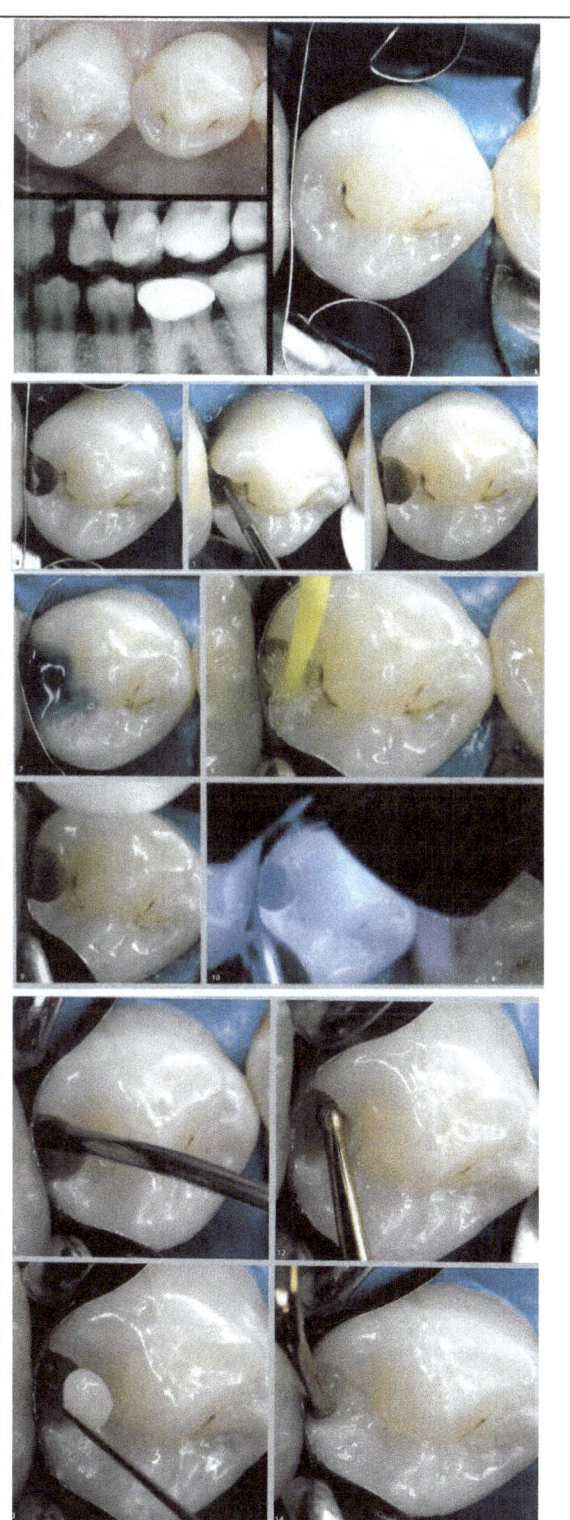

Isolation: Dental Rubber Dam and a metal interproximal guard (InterGuard, Ultradent)
Material: A2-shaded flowable composite (Grandio Flow, Voco)
The instrument used for uniformly distributing the material: a ball-tipped instrument (M-1 Ball Burnisher XP)
Material for successive increments: a 02-shaded opacious hybrid composite (Amaris, Voco)
An instrument for condensing increments: A ball-tipped instrument is used for increment
The final enamel layer: a neutral translucency (Amaris NT, Voco),
While the material was still soft an invagination was made with a 08 endodontic file (K-Flex, SybronEndo).
Initial finish: with a silicone carbide impregnated brush that removes any remaining surface defects
The final polish of the occlusal surface of the direct restoration was rendered with a synthetic foam cup, aluminum oxide paste, and the incremental use of water

CLASS IV COMPOSITE RESTORATION

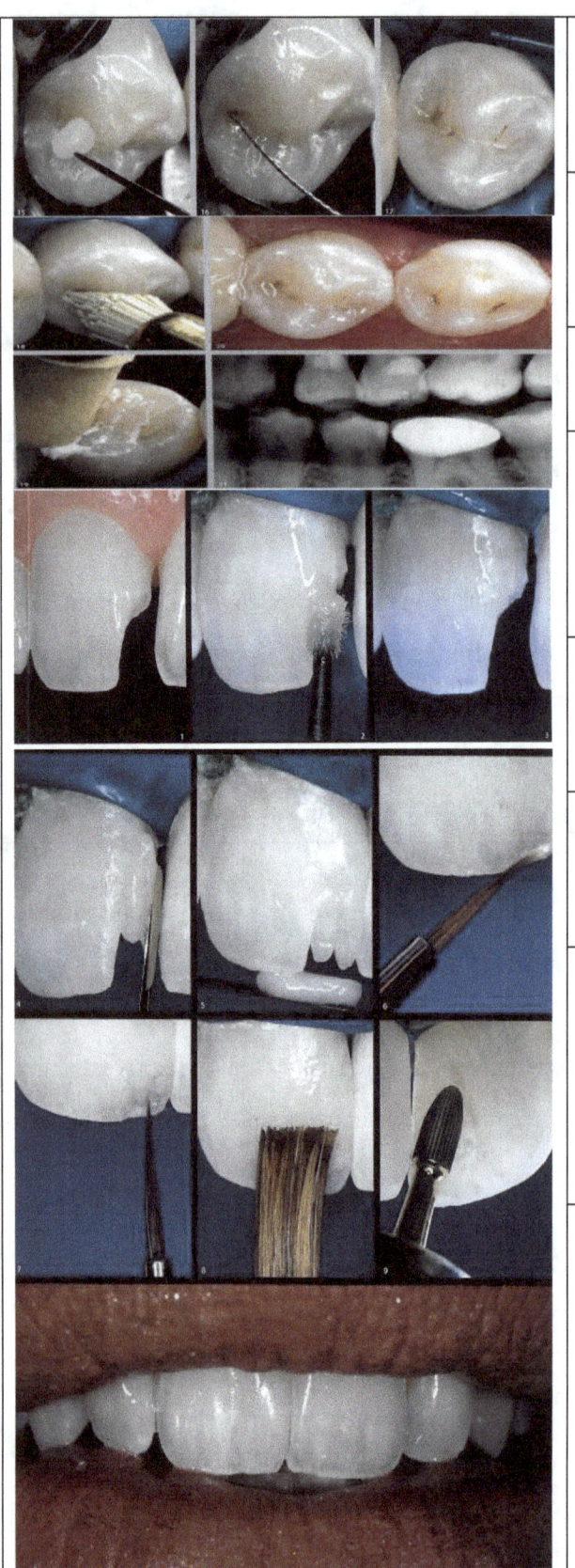

A light-cured adhesive (OptiBond Solo Plus, Kerr/Sybron) was applied with a disposable applicator
The first layer of the dentin body: a B1-shaded hybrid composite resin (Point 4, Kerr/Sybron)
Contoured, and smoothed: using an artist's #4 sable brush
An elongated increment of XL1-shaded hybrid composite resin (Point 4), was applied to the inciso-lingual and contoured to form an incisal matrix
A diluted white tint (Kolor + Plus, Kerr/Sybron) was placed along the horizontal invagination and light cured for 40 second
A diluted blue tint (Kolor + Plus) was placed in the vertical invaginations to create an illusion of translucency
The final artificial enamel layer, a translucent shaded hybrid composite resin applied, adapted, and smoothed into an ideal anatomical contour with a #4 artist's sable brush
To refine the lingual anatomy, a #30-fluted egg-shaped finishing bur was used with light pressure to prevent heating of the build-up done.

COMPOSITE CLASS V RESTORATION

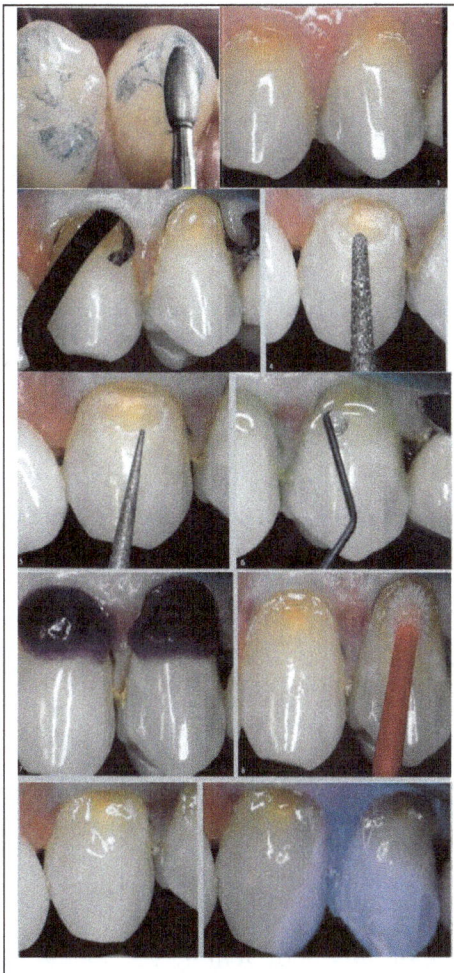	Gingival retraction: Gingival retraction cord used to access gingival margin
	Margin: A chamfer bur used to place a chamfer margin along the occlusal margin
	The preparations were scrubbed with a slurry mixture of disinfectant (Consepsis, Ultradent) and pumice
	Application of adhesive: A thin tipped Applicator tip
	Material: The dentin layer, an A1 /B1-shaded hybrid composite (Synergy D6), was applied to the occlusal half of the preparation, second layer of hybrid composite (Synergy D6), followed by universal enamel-shaded hybrid composite (Synergy D6)
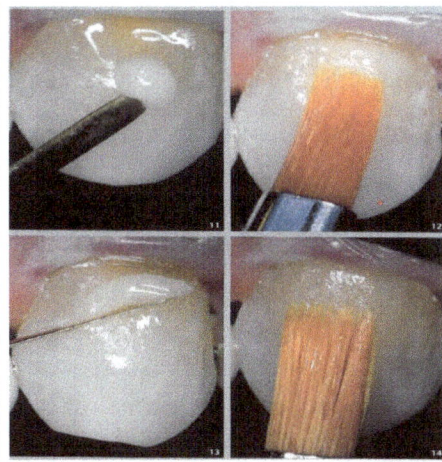	Contouring: with a long-bladed composite instrument
	Each incremental layer was smoothed with a #2 artist sable brush to prevent surface irregularities

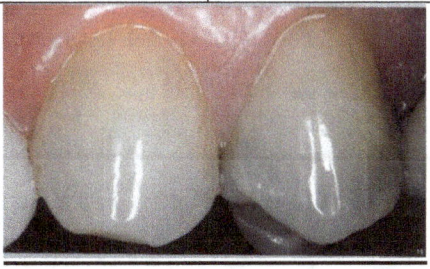

REFERENCES

1. **Phillips RW, Avery DR, Mehra R, Swartz ML, McCune RJ.** Observations on a composite resin for Class II restorations: Two-year report. J Prosthet Dent 1972; 28:164-169.

2. **Phillips RW, Avery DR, Mehra R, Swartz ML, McCune RJ.** Observations on a composite resin for Class II restorations: Three-year report. J Prosthet Dent 1973; 30:891-897.

3. **Lutz F, Phillips RW, Roulet JF, Setcos JC.** In vivo and in vitro wear of potential posterior composites. J Dent Res 1984; 63:914-920.

4. **Leinfelder KF, Sluder TB, Santos JF, Wall JT.** Five-year clinical evaluation of anterior and posterior restorations of composite resin. Oper Dent 1980; 5:57-65.

5. **Leinfelder KF, Roberson TM.** Clinical evaluation of posterior composite resins. Gen Dent 1983; 31:276-280.

6. **Rubinstein S, Nidetz AJ.** Posterior direct resin-bonded restorations: Still an esthetic alternative. J Esthet Dent 1995; 7:167—173.

7. **Jackson RD, Morgan M.** The new posterior resins and a simplified placement technique. J Am Dent Assoc 2000; 31:375—383.

8. **Bichacho N.** Direct composite resin restorations of the anterior single tooth: Clinical implications and practical applications. Compend Contin Educ Dent 1996; 17:796-802.

9. **Dietschi D, Scampa U, Campanile G, Holz J.** Marginal adaptation and seal of direct and indirect Class II composite resin restorations: An in vitro evaluation. Quintessence Int 1995; 26:127-138. 10.

10. **Full CA, Hollander WR.** The composite resin restoration: A literature review. Part I: Proper cavity preparation and placement techniques. ASDC J Dent Child 1993; 60:48-51.

11. **Dietschi D, De Siebentha! G, Neveu-Rosenstand L, Holz J.** Influence of the restorative technique and new adhesives on the dentin marginal seal and adaptation of resin composite Glass II restorations: An in vitro evaluation. Quintessence Int 1995; 26:717-727.

12. **Eames WB, Strain JD, Weitman RT, Williams AK.** Clinical comparison of composite, amalgam, and silicate restorations. J Am Dent Assoc 1974; 89:1111-1117.

13. **Mazik CA.** Simplified occlusal anatomy for posterior composites. J Esthet Dent 1992; 4:8-10.
14. **Ruyter IE.** Composites—Characterization of composite filling materials: Reactor response. Adv Dent Res 1988; 2:122-129. 15.
15. **Hornbrook DS.** Optimizing form and function with the direct posterior composite resin: A case report. Pract Periodontics Aesthet Dent 1996; 8:405-411. 16.
16. **Dickerson WG.** A functional and aesthetic direct resin technique. Pract Periodontics Aesthet Dent 1991; 3:43-47. 17.
17. **Leinfelder KF.** A conservative approach to placing posterior composite resin restorations. J Am Dent Assoc 1996; 127:743-748. 18.
18. **Mazer RB, Leinfelder KF.** Evaluating a microfill posterior composite resin: A five-year study. J Am Dent Assoc 1992; 123:32-38. 22.
19. **Mazer RB, Leinfelder KF.** Clinical evaluation of a posterior composite resin containing a new type of filler. J Esthet Dent 1988; 1:66-70. 23.
20. **Dickinson GL, Gerbo LR, Leinfelder KF.** Clinical evaluation of a highly wear-resistant com- posite. Am J Dent 1993; 6:85-87. 24.
21. **Wendt SL Jr, Leinfelder KF.** Clinical evaluation of Clearfil Photoposterior: 3-year results. Am J Dent 1992; 5:121-125.
22. **Roberson TM, Heymann HO, Swift JR.** Sturdevant's Art and Science of Operative Dentistry, ed 4. St Louis: Mosby, 2002.
23. **Lee SM.** Preface to the Dictionary of Composite Material Technology. Lancaster, PA: Tech-nomic, 1989.
24. **Talib R.** Dental composites: A review. J Nihon Univ Sch Dent 1993; 35:161-170.
25. **Ferracane JL.** Current trends in dental composites. Crit Rev Oral Biol Med 1995; 6:302—318. 30.
26. **Albers HF.** Tooth-Colored Restoratives: Principles and Techniques, ed 9. Hamilton, ON: BC Decker, 2002. 31.
27. **Iga M, Takeshige F, UiT, Torii M.** The relationship between polymerization shrinkage measured by a modified dilatometer and the inorganic filler content of light-cured composites. Dent Mater J 1991; 10:38-45. 32.
28. **Munksgaard EC, Hansen EK, Kato H.** Wall-to-wall polymerization contraction of composite resins versus filler content. Scand J Dent Res 1987; 95:526-531.
29. **Soderholm KJ.** Influence of silane treatment and filler fraction on thermal expansion of composite resins. J Dent Res 1984; 63:1321-1326.

30. **Bowen RL.** Properties of a silica-reinforced polymer for dental restorations. J Am Dent As- soc 1963; 66:57-64.
31. **Hosoda H, Yamada T, Inokoshi S.** SEM and elemental analysis of composite resins. J Pros- thet Dent 1990; 64:669-676. 36.
32. **Van Dijken JW, Wing KR, Ruyter IE.** An evaluation of the radiopacity of composite restorative materials used in Class I and Class II cavities. Acta Odontol Scand 1989; 47:401-407.
33. **Roulet JF.** Degradation of Dental Polymers. Basel: S. Karger AG, 1987.
34. **Davidson CL, Feilzer AJ.** Polymerization shrinkage and polymerization shrinkage stress in polymer-based restoratives. J Dent 1997; 25:435-440. 47.
35. **Venhoven BA, de Gee AJ, Davidson CL.** Polymerization contraction and conversion of light-curing BisGMA-based methacrylate resins. Biomaterials 1993; 14:871-875.
36. **Ouellet D.** Considerations and techniques for multiple bulk-fill direct posterior compos- ites. Compendium 1995; 16:1212-1224. 49.
37. **Feilzer AJ, de Gee AJ,Davidson CL.** Setting stress in composite resin in relation to the configuration of the restoration. J Dent Res 1987; 66:1636-1639. 50.
38. **Feilzer AJ,Dooren LH, de Gee AJ,Davidson CL.** Influence of light intensity on polymerization shrinkage and integrity of restoration-cavity interface. Euro J Oral Sci 1995; 103:322- 326.
39. **Kemp-Scholte CM, Davidson CL.** Complete marginal seal of Class V resin composite restorations affected by increased flexibility. J Dent Res 1990; 69:1240—1243
40. **Terry DA.** Natural Aesthetics with Composite Resin. Mahwah, NJ: Montage Media, 2004.
41. **Asmussen E.** Composite restorative resins. Composition versus wall-to-wall polymerization contraction. Acta Odontol Scand 1975; 33:337-343.
42. **Unterbrink GL, Muessner R.** Influence of light intensity on two restorative systems. J Dent 1995; 23:183-189. 54.
43. **Uno S, Asmussen E.** Marginal adaptation of a restorative resin polymerized at a reduced rate. Scand J Dent Res 1991; 99:440-444.
44. Top 10 Composite & Plastic Filling Instruments | Dental Country™ https://www.pattersondental.com/Supplies/ItemDetail/073939758

45. **N. Walther,** OptraSculpt Handlingstest, Test Report, Ivoclar, 2016 [2]
46. **L. Enggist,** Use Validation OptraFoam Extension, Test Report, Ivoclar, 2017 [3]
47. **A. Peschke, S. Heintze,** Design valid ierungstestbericht OptraFoam, Test Report, Ivoclar, 2012

CHAPTER-6
BIOMODIFICATION OF TOOTH DISCOLORATIONS

Ask the average person how they would most like to improve their smile and the answer would often be "with whiter and brighter teeth." It is commonly known that people are responded more positively when they have a dazzling, healthy smile.

Most newly formed teeth have thick, even enamel. This enamel layer modifies the base color of the underlying dentin, creating a milky white appearance.[1] For many of your patients, that bright, white look can typify youth, health, and physical attractiveness. It is the look against which they measure the appearance of their teeth. For some, unfortunately, their teeth will seem dingy and discolored in comparison. Teeth become stained and discolored, sometimes before they even erupt, almost always as they age, for one or more genetic, environmental, medical, or dental reasons. The most common problems are the superficial color changes that result from tobacco, coffee, tea, or highly colored foods. Teeth that contain microcracks are particularly susceptible to these stains. Discoloration also occurs through the penetration of the tooth structure by a discoloring agent, such as a medication given systemically, excessive fluoride ingested during the development of tooth enamel, by-products of the body such as bilirubin released into the dentinal tubules during illness, trauma (primarily the breakdown of hemoglobin), or pigmentation from the medicaments and materials used in dental repair. Wear and thinning of the enamel caused by aging, too abrasive cleaning materials, aggressive brushing, and acidic food and drink also can diminish the covering power of the white enamel, letting more of the darker-hued dentin show through.[1]

Severe discoloration of a tooth or teeth can be a major esthetic problem. For the appropriate patient, with careful diagnosis, case selection, treatment planning, and attention to technique, bleaching can be the simplest, least invasive, and least expensive approach to brighter teeth. Sometimes one office session is sufficient to change a patient's appearance dramatically. If considered an adjunct to other procedures for correcting discoloration and other esthetic problems, bleaching extends the promise to an even larger group of patients seeking more attractive teeth. This chapter will provide current concepts and the latest scientific evidence in tooth bleaching that can fulfill our patient's desire for a whiter and brighter smile.

BLEACHING VITAL TEETH

The earliest efforts to bleach teeth go back more than a century and focused on the search for an effective bleaching agent to paint on discolored teeth.

Zaragoza,[2] Abbot had introduced by 1918 the forerunner of the combination used to bleach vital teeth today: hydrogen peroxide and an accelerated reaction caused by devices delivering heat to the teeth. In the early 1960s, Goldstein developed the first commercial bleaching light for the in-office bleaching of vital teeth.

In the 1970s when a growing number of dentists saw how well it worked on the stains caused by tetracycline ingestion at critical developmental stages of the teeth. Although many of the mechanisms by which bleaching removes discoloration may not be fully understood, the basic process almost certainly involves oxidation, during which the molecules causing the discoloration are released. The use of heat and light devices appears to accelerate the oxidation reaction.[3,4] For the next 20 years, in-office bleaching or power bleaching by dentists proved helpful for this and other problems.

In the early 1990s, bleaching gained new prominence in the public eye by introducing and aggressively marketing bleaching materials intended to be used without dental evaluation and monitoring.[5] The widespread acceptance of these products can also be seen as a disturbing trend due to the potential for misdiagnosis, use of bleaching for inappropriate conditions, poorly fitting mouthguards, and unesthetic or painful results. Bleaching materials applied inappropriately may make the existing situation worse, creating uneven color change or deleteriously affecting restorations. The availability of such products places additional responsibility on the dental profession to make people aware of how well professionally applied bleaching works, or whether it works at all, depends on the discoloration itself, its cause, the length of time the discoloring agent has permeated the structure of the tooth, and other factors about which a dentist's advice and monitoring are critical.

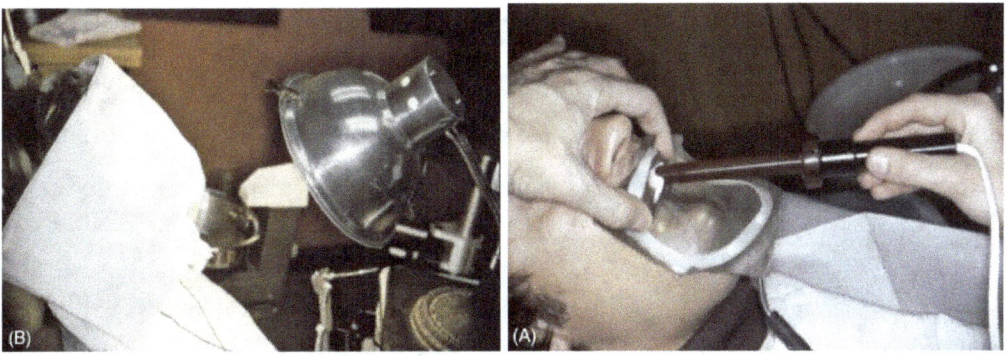

FIGURE 6.1 (A) In the early 1960s, Christensen showed individual teeth bleaching using a modified soldering iron.

(B) Also in the 1960s, Goldstein showed in-office bleaching using a modified photoflood lamp to bleach multiple teeth.

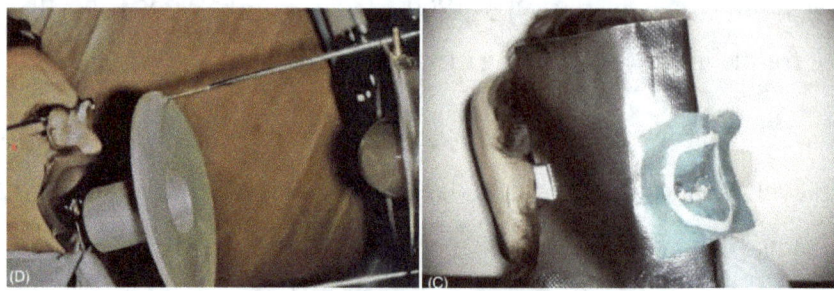

FIGURE 16.1 (C) Due to the excessive heat created by the photoflood lamp, Goldstein developed a bleaching shield that protected the patient's face.

(D) Goldstein later modified the bleaching light to better isolate the heat and light into a narrower zone for bleaching individual teeth.

A good visual examination usually will suggest the etiology of discoloration and consequently the appropriateness of bleaching as a treatment. The diagnostic workup should include pre-treatment photographs, X-ray films, and intensive prophylaxis to remove superficial staining that may be compounding more intrinsic discoloration.

ETIOLOGY OF DISCOLORATION

A) **Extrinsic stains**: caused by the accumulation of stains on the enamel surface and can be accentuated by pitting or irregularities of the enamel, salivary composition, salivary flow rates, and poor oral hygiene.[6] Various types of discoloration ranging from orange, green, brown, and black can be observed and are mostly a result of highly colored beverages or food. e associated with chromogenic bacteria which can be easily removed by dental prophylaxis. Nicotine stains start as tenacious extrinsic stains, but over time absorb into the tooth and become intrinsic stains that tend to be more difficult to bleach.[7] Drug-related tooth discoloration can be either extrinsic or intrinsic. The most common drugs causing extrinsic discoloration include chlorhexidine[8] oral iron salts in liquid form, essential oils,[9] and co-amoxiclav.[10]

B) **Intrinsic stains**: Unlike extrinsic discolorations that can be more easily removed by prophylaxis and bleaching, intrinsic discolorations are due to stain molecules within the enamel and dentin, incorporated either during tooth formation or after the eruption.[11] Dental fluorosis is the most common cause of intrinsic discoloration because of the wide range of availability from multiple sources.[12] Clinically, fluorosis presents as localized areas of white, yellow, or orange discolorations and in severe cases is accompanied by surface pitting or severe surface defects.[6] Bleaching is a good indication of fluorosis with brown pigmentation on a smooth enamel surface.

C) **Tetracycline stain**: The success of bleaching for the yellow or brown stains caused by tetracycline discoloration was key to its place in the emerging field of dental esthetics. The devastating effect on tooth formation of as little as 1g of tetracycline was recognized in the late 1950s,[13] with the first certain identification reported by a study of cystic fibrosis patients by **Shwachman et al.**[14] In 1970, **Cohen and Parkins** published a method for bleaching the discolored dentin of young adults with cystic fibrosis who had undergone tetracycline treatment.[15] The results were promising, and dentists concerned with esthetics began applying bleaching procedures to other stains and discolorations.

D) **Stain from dental conditions or treatments**: Dental caries are a primary cause of pigmentation and may be seen as an opaque, white halo, or gray discoloration. An even deeper brown-to-black discoloration can result from bacterial degradation of food debris in areas of tooth decay or decomposing fillings. Such problems should be corrected before bleaching. Restorations also frequently cause discolorations. Degraded tooth-colored restorations such as acrylics, glass ionomers, or composites can cause teeth to look grayer and discolored. Metal restorations, such as amalgams, even silver, and gold, can reflect discoloration through the enamel and should be replaced with less visible materials such as composite resin before bleaching.[16] Oils, iodines, nitrates, root canal sealers, pins, and other materials used in dental restorations can cause discoloration. The length of time these substances have been allowed to penetrate the dentinal tubules will determine the amount of residual discoloration and will, consequently, affect the success of bleaching. Metallic stains are the most difficult to remove. Endodontic materials and sealers have various staining potentials that cause intrinsic discoloration of the root canal-filled tooth over time.

E) **Stain from systemic conditions**: Developmental defects of enamel or dentin can be associated with amelogenesis imperfecta, dentinogenesis imperfecta, and enamel hypoplasia. Amelogenesis imperfecta is a hereditary disorder of enamel formation involving both the primary and permanent dentition.[17] Discolorations associated with amelogenesis imperfecta tend to aggravate with time as the rough surfaces allow stains to accumulate more easily. Dentinogenesis imperfecta is a hereditary disorder affecting both dentitions, exhibiting abnormal dentin formation. Affected teeth exhibit slender roots, small or obliterated pulp chambers, and root canals with enamel that easily chip away from the dentin.[18] Enamel hypoplasia is the incomplete or defective formation of the enamel matrix induced by systemic or local factors. Hematologic disorders cause the deposition of blood pigments in the dentin or enamel resulting in discoloration of the tooth structure. Bleaching can be quite effective for the discoloration caused by infusion of the dentin during development.

- The bluish-green or brown primary teeth seen in children who suffered severe jaundice as infants. The stains are the result of postnatal staining of the dentin by bilirubin or biliverdin.
- The characteristically brownish teeth caused by the destruction of an excessive number of erythrocytes in the blood cells that occurs in erythroblastosis fetalis, a result of Rhesus factor incompatibility between mother and fetus.
- The purplish-brown teeth color of persons with porphyria, an extremely rare condition that causes excess production of pigment.

F) **Discoloration due to aging**: With the aging population, an increasing number of your patients will be older. Most persons in our youth-oriented society easily accept the changes in color, form, and texture of teeth that almost inevitably accompany aging. The type and degree of such changes will depend on a mixture of genetics, use and abuse, and habits. Years of smoking and coffee drinking have a cumulative staining effect, and these and other stains become even more visible because of the inevitable cracking and other changes on the surface of the tooth, within its crystalline structure, and in the underlying dentin and pulp. In addition to wear and trauma on the teeth, amalgams and other restorations placed years ago may begin to degrade. Even with the most careful avoidance of or attention to such problems, our teeth are likely to become more discolored as we age, from both natural wear and exposure to normal environmental contaminants. The first change to occur is usually a thinning of the enamel. This may cause the facial surface of the tooth to appear flat with a progressive shift in color due to a loss of the translucent enamel layer. At the same time, the enamel begins to thin, and secondary dentin formation begins through a natural tooth-protective mechanism in the dentin and pulp. For many of the discolorations seen in older patients, home matrix bleaching can be a safe, effective treatment option. Additionally, unless the enamel is too badly worn, in-office or combined bleaching can be an effective treatment. For many older patients, the short time required in the dental chair, relatively low cost, and lack of trauma involved, make bleaching an especially appealing treatment.

CONTRAINDICATIONS TO BLEACHING OF VITAL TEETH USING IN-OFFICE TECHNIQUES

There are as follows:

- Extremely large pulps, which may increase sensitivity.
- Other causes of hypersensitivity, such as exposed root surfaces or the transient hyperemia associated with orthodontic tooth movement.
- Severe loss of enamel due to attrition, abrasion, or erosion
- Teeth exhibiting gross or microscopic enamel cracking
- Extremely dark teeth, and severe tetracycline staining, especially those with marked banding
- Teeth with white or opaque spots: although bleaching will not eradicate these spots, the process can lighten the surrounding tooth structure and then the white spots can be eliminated with micro-abrasion or with bonding
- Teeth in which some restorations must be matched or, especially, teeth that have been bonded or veneered
- Extensive restorations
- Patients who are perfectionists: bleaching is not perfect, in the way veneers can be. This is especially true for severe stains. With darker tetracycline stains, for example, the majority of the bleaching will occur on the incisal one-half of the teeth. The remaining surfaces can only be partially helped by a selective bleaching solution and heat application.

Techniques for in-office bleaching of vital teeth

In-office whitening provides an alternative to home bleaching, especially when patients desire faster results and demonstrate low compliance in wearing a tray at home. In-office whitening can be performed on selective teeth, on one arch, or even on both arches where speedy treatment is desired. Generally, the whitening effect is noticed immediately after a single session. However, generally, a single session is not enough to achieve optimal results and for maximum bleaching, several appointments are required.

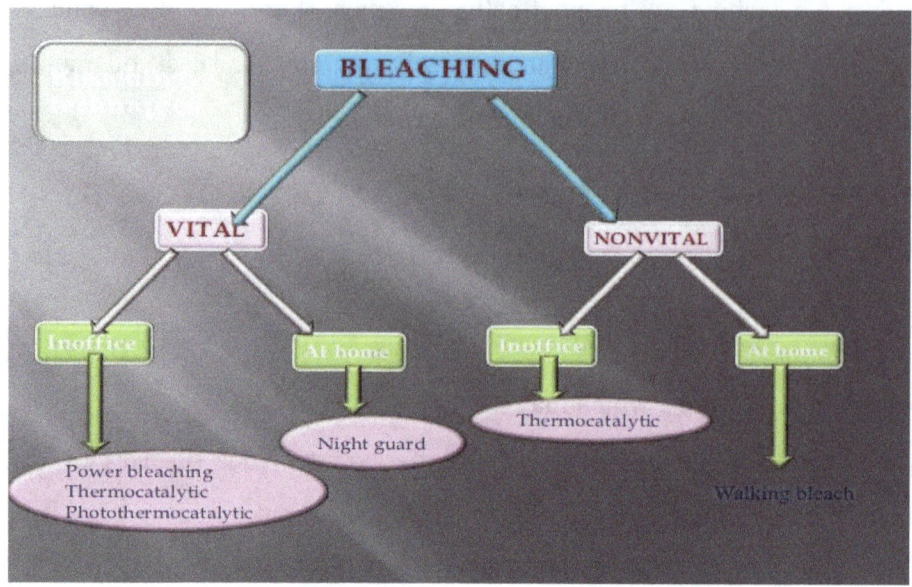

PREPARATION AND APPLICATION OF BLEACHING MATERIAL

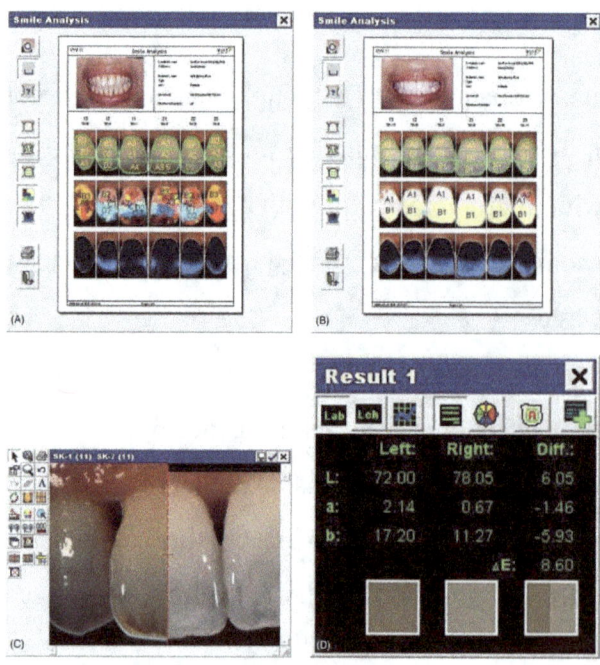

FIGURE 6.2: (A–C) The benefit of using complete tooth measurement devices in tooth bleaching is the ability to print out before and after smile analyses that can effectively motivate the patient into the treatment. The before and after images can also be synchronized. (D) Measuring the color change as expressed as ΔE

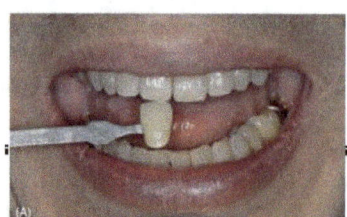

FIGURE 6.3: (A) A shade guide is used to record the baseline color.

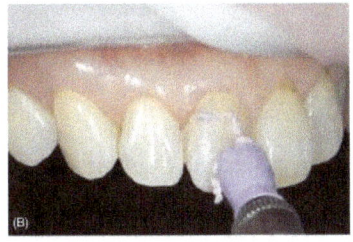

(B) Polishing kit: used to free the teeth of all surface stains and plaque.

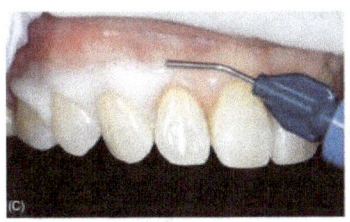 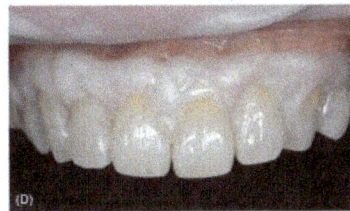

(C, D) A resin barrier (Opal Dam, Ultradent): to cover the cervical area of the tooth and extend onto the gingiva.

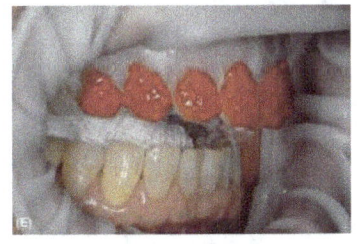

(E) A highly concentrated bleaching applied material homogeneously onto the tooth (Opalescence Boost, Ultradent).

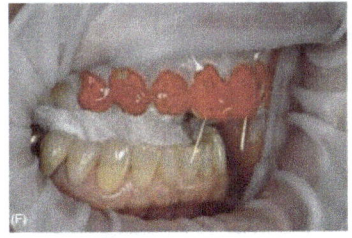

(F) A precut linear low-density polyethylene wrap (Saran wrap): placed onto the teeth to prevent evaporation of the active material and create a good seal.

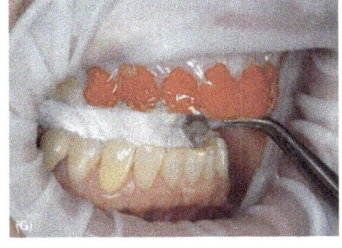 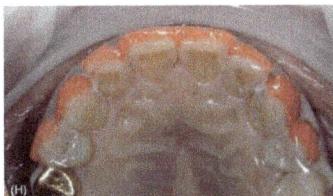

(G, H) Cotton pliers: used to seal the wrap around the incisal edges.

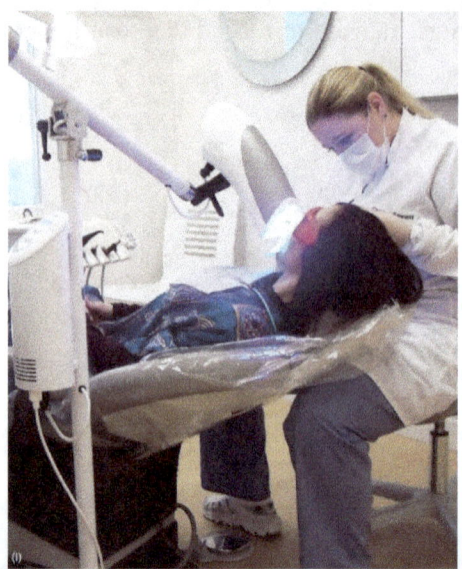
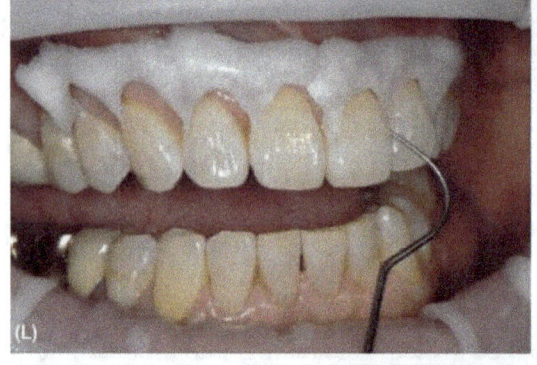
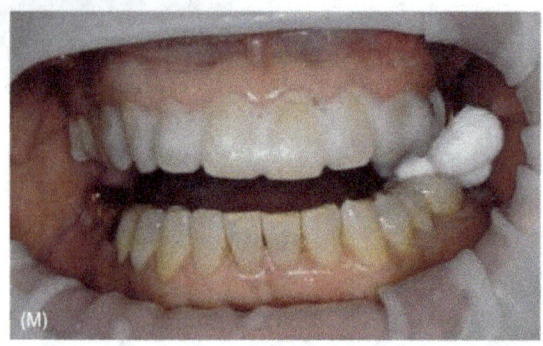
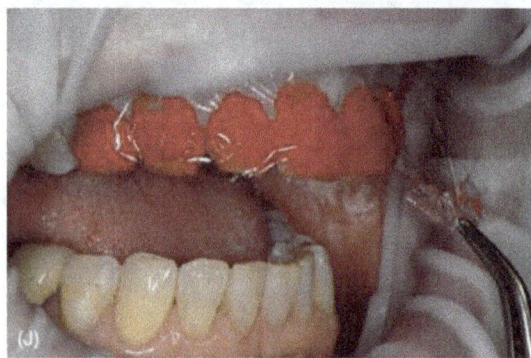
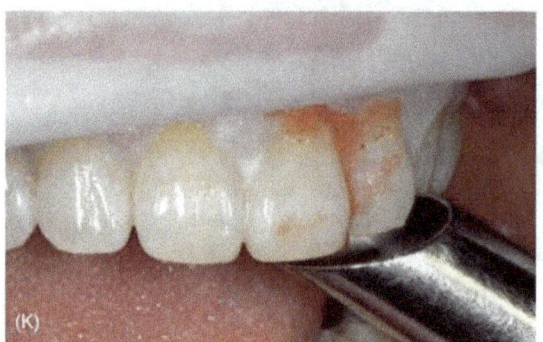

FIGURE 6.2 (I) Bleaching Unit: activation of bleaching material

(J, K, L) Remove the resin barrier with the explorer tip.

(M) 2% neutral sodium fluoride gel for finishing.

Matrix bleaching (nightguard vital bleaching)

Matrix bleaching refers to bleaching procedures that the patient uses outside the dental office. Wearing a matrix fabricated by the dentist, the patient can apply a bleaching material to the affected teeth while at his or her office, exercise facility, driving a car, or almost any place in daily life.

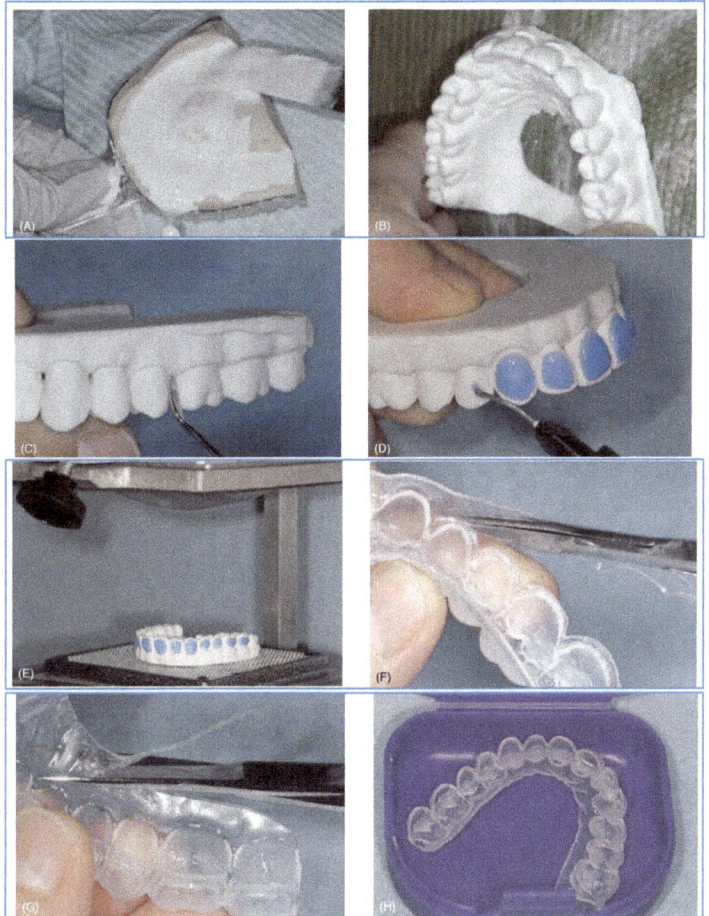

FIGURE 6.3: (A) An alginate impression of the arch to be treated is made, and stone is poured carefully to avoid any bubble or void formation

(B) The stone model is trimmed so that the base is flat and parallel to the occlusal plane.

(C) The gingival margin on the stone model is redefined with a sharp instrument to create a better seal around the tray margin.

(D) A thin layer of block-out resin can be placed on the buccal surface as a reservoir for the bleaching material.

(E) A soft and thin sheet is heated in a vacuum-forming unit until it sags 12mm.

(F) The tray is trimmed with sharp scissors approximately 0.5mm away from the gingival margin to create a scalloped pattern on the buccal surface.

(G) The lingual border is extended 2mm from the gingival margin in a straight pattern.

(H) The finished tray is cleaned and stored in a tray case until delivery to the patient.

INSIDE-OUTSIDE TRAY BLEACHING TECHNIQUE

This technique was described by **Settembrini and Liebenberg** [18] in 1997 to bleach the discolored tooth from the inside as well as from the outside with a 10% carbamide peroxide solution retained in a custom-fitted tray. The major advantage of this technique is that the nonvital discolored tooth can be bleached together with the adjacent vital teeth.

1. Deliver a custom-fitted tray and 10% carbamide peroxide solution to the patient.

2. Give instructions on how to insert the bleaching gel into the cavity and the tray.

3. Show the patient how to clean the open-access cavity with the use of an empty syringe.

4. Have the patient return to the office, once the teeth have whitened.

Out-of-office bleaching technique (or walking bleach)

Follow the same preparation techniques given earlier.

1. On a glass mixing slab, prepare a bleaching paste of peroxy borate monohydrate (Amosan) or sodium perborate and enough 35% hydrogen peroxide to form a thick white paste.

2. Fill the entire preparation with the bleaching paste, leaving adequate space to place a temporary restoration and sealer. Make certain that the seal is effective as the moist paste can damage tissue if it leaks into the pulp chamber. One method is to carefully apply a solvent (Prep Dry, PrimaDry [Ultradent]) around the enamel margin and flow a medium-stiff mix of Cavit to close the area. If the patient experiences a burning on the tongue, rinse until the sensation is gone.

3. Have the patient return in 3–5 days. If the degree of bleaching is not sufficient, repeat the entire procedure. Again, a slight overbleaching is desirable since teeth tend to darken slightly after the final bleach.

Finishing

1. Remove the cotton or bleaching paste and swab the preparation throughout with acetone or xylol.

2. Air dry internally and throughout the bleached crown to penetrate and seal the dentinal tubules and maintain the tooth's translucency. Use several coats of a clear dentin bonding agent to prevent recurrent coronal stains.

3. Etch the marginal walls with 35% phosphoric acid to assure good mechanical bonding. The entire restoration is placed at one time and finished properly to assure good marginal adaptation.

4. Apply a dental bonding agent and cure before filling the cavity with composite resin restorative materials of the lightest shade aesthetically compatible with the tooth. Use a composite with a good dentin bonding agent, being careful to etch the enamel walls before restoring the final area. A micro-fill or polishable hybrid is the best material to use because it allows a polished surface to blend with the adjacent enamel surface.

MAINTAINING BLEACHING RESULTS

Although both in-office and matrix techniques can produce effective results, the advantage of the latter technique is that it will allow for touch-ups or retreatment as necessary. As long as the matrix continues to fit properly, a new solution can be given to the patient for an additional series of bleaching treatments every few years or as needed. Generally, it may be 3 years before retreatment is desirable.[19, 20]

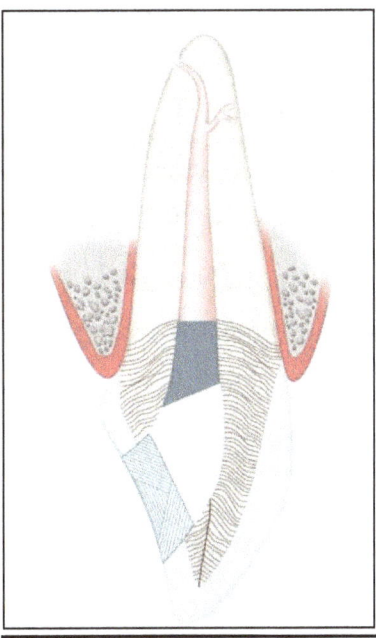

FIGURE 6.4: The walking bleach requires an effective seal for the bleaching paste to remain active.

REFERENCES

1. **Dzierzak J.** Factors that cause tooth color changes protocol for in-office "power" bleaching. Pract Periodontics Aesthet Dent 1991;3(2):15–20.

2. **Zaragoza VMT.** Bleaching of vital teeth: technique. Estomodeo 1984; 9:7–30.

3. Friedman J. Variability of lamp characteristics in dental curing lights. J Esthet Dent 1989;1(6):189–190.

4. **Hodosh M, Mirman M, Shklar G, Povar M.** A new method of bleaching discolored teeth by the use of a solid-state direct heating device. Dent Dig 1970;76(8):344–346.

5. **Haywood VB.** The Food and drug administration and its Influence on home bleaching. Curr Opin Cosmet Dent 1993:12–18.

6. **Hattab FN, Qudeimat MA, Al-Rimawi HS.** Dental discoloration: an overview. J Esthet Dent 1999; 11:291–310.

7. **Haywood United States, IL. VB.** Tooth Whitening: Indications and Outcomes of Nightguard Vital Bleaching. Chicago, IL: Quintessence; 2007.

8. **Addy M, Roberts WR.** Comparison of the bis-biguanide antiseptics alexidine and chlorhexidine. II. clinical and in vitro staining properties. J Clin Periodontol 1981;8(3):220–230.

9. **Addy M, Moran J, Newcombe R, Warren P.** The comparative tea staining potential of phenolic, chlorhexidine, and anti-adhesive mouth rinses. J Clin Periodontol 1995;22(12):923–928.

10. **Garcia-Lopez M, Martinez-Blanco M, Martinez-Mir I, Palop V.** Amoxycillin-clavulanic acid-related tooth discoloration in children. Pediatrics 2001;108(3):81

11. **Dahl JE, Palleson U.** Tooth bleaching: a critical review of the biological aspects. Crit Rev Oral Biol Med 2003;14(4):292–304.

12. **Burt BA.** The changing patterns of systemic fluoride intake. J Dent Res 1992;71(5):1228–1237.

13. **Arens D.** The role of bleaching in esthetics. Dent Clin North Am 1989;33(2):319–336.

14. **Shwachman H, Fekete E, Kulezychi L, Foley G.** The effect of long-term antibiotic therapy in patients with cystic fibrosis of the pancreas. Antibiot Annu 1958–1959;6:692–699.

15. **Cohen S, Parkins FM.** Bleaching tetracycline-stained vital teeth. Oral Surg Oral Med Oral Pathol 1970;29(3):465–471.

16. **Bailey SJ, Swift EJ Jr.** Effects of home bleaching products on composite resins. Quintessence Int 1992;23(7):489–494.
17. **Stewart RE, Witkop CJ, Bixler D.** Pediatric Dentistry: Scientific Foundations and Clinical Practice. St Louis, MO: C.V. Mosby; 1982.
18. **Faunce F.** Management of discolored teeth. Dent Clin North Am 1983;27(4):657–670.
19. **Haywood VB.** Achieving, maintaining, and recovering successful tooth bleaching. J Esthet Dent 1996;8(1):31–38.
20. **Kwon S, Ko S, Greenwall L.** Tooth Whitening in Esthetic Dentistry. Germany: Quintessence; 2009.

CHAPTER-7
TOOTH PREPARATIONS

In 1881, **M. H. Webb** demonstrated a concept of preparation whereby the margins of enamel were free from contact with the adjacent tooth, preventing the extension of decay and promoting cleansing by saliva and fluids ingested into the oral cavity.[1, 2] In this same timeline, **G. V. Black** introduced the phrase "extension for prevention",[3, 4] indicating that by extending the preparation to the proximal line angle, the margins of the restoration would be self-cleansing by way of food excursion. His concept also included extending preparations through enamel fissures to allow Cavosurface margins to be placed on non-fissured enamel.[5] These principles of cavity preparation were designed for use with metallic restorative materials, and these non-adhesive materials required preparations with resistance and retention geometric forms.

These concepts of the "mechanical era" sanctioned the removal of healthy, sound tooth structures to retain the restorative material.[4] The preparation dimensions were designed to overcome the restorative material's limited mechanical characteristics (i.e., fracture resistance). At that time, operative dentistry combined the need to eliminate caries with the requirements to prepare the tooth to accommodate the properties of the restorative materials in use.[4]

The available restorative materials were designed only to obturate the cavity and were non-adhesive and thus could not seal the restorative interface. In addition, they were not bioactive and could not arrest or eliminate caries. When **GV Black** proposed these principles and his classification of cavity designs, the industry focused on controlling rampant caries. Unfortunately, this focus was not based on scientific knowledge of the disease or on any scientific rationale.[6, 7] By the middle of the twentieth century, clinicians challenged existing principles using more conservative preparations in an attempt to preserve the maximum integrity of the natural tooth structure.[1-7] The last half of the twentieth century introduced adhesive surface preparation of the enamel and dentin (i.e., acid etching and self-etching) and composite resin technology, which allowed for more conservative preparations without a standard geometric form.[1] "Prevention from extension" seeks to minimize the biological cost of the natural tooth as a whole [8-9] by adopting a philosophy that combines prevention, remineralization, and minimal intervention for the replacement of natural tooth structure or restorations.[10] In the past, cavity preparation was designed in an attempt to arrest the caries process. These ideas were based on the removal of caries and the mechanical properties of the filling materials in use to treat them.[11] At the time, neither the fluoride ion nor the process of remineralization was known.[8] In the new era of "prevention from extension, "many of the old limitations are no longer applicable because of advances in research and technology. Increased patient awareness, superior diagnostic capabilities (i.e., enhanced vision and illumination), and improvements in biomaterials and instruments have all contributed to a more conservative approach to tooth preparation.[12]

CLINICAL OBJECTIVES OF MODERN RESTORATIVE DENTISTRY

From the onset of disease to the initial placement of the restoration, the clinical objectives of contemporary restorative dentistry are Prevention, Preservation, And Conservation.

A) **PREVENTION:** The primary objective of the clinician is to prevent the placement of the initial restoration.[13] Prevention begins with contemporary restorative procedures such as remineralization, sealants, and preventive resin restorations that require less invasive procedures. The introduction of these minimally invasive procedures in conjunction with preventive measures such as dietary modifications, frequent professional plaque control, fluoride administration, specific antimicrobial treatment, and improved oral hygiene through patient education may reduce dental caries. This preventive approach provides the patient and the clinician with an opportunity to re-evaluate the outcome of the preventive measures and possibly reduce the potential for invasive intervention.[14]

B) **PRESERVATION:** The second clinical objective of contemporary restorative dentistry is to preserve tooth structure during preparation for restoration. The preservation of natural tooth structure begins with the elimination of disease, followed by remineralization and healing of demineralized areas. This process may be applied to minimal-intervention procedures, replacement restorations, and the repair of enlarged cavities. Adhesive preparation designs should be based on the conservation of tooth structure, using adhesive bioactive restorative material.[15, 16]

C) **CONSERVATION:** The conservative concept of adhesive tooth preparation requires a biologic approach,[17] which represents a key component of adhesive dentistry.[18] Adhesive restorative materials have a greater potential for bonding to the tooth structure, while metallic restorations require mechanical retention. The enamel has a significant contribution to the retention and strength of the restoration provided that the enamel is strong, completely mineralized, and well-supported by dentin. The incorporation of bevels provides union at the ends of the enamel rods instead of at their long axis, which increases surface area, provides strength, and increases retention.[13]

The adhesive restoration does not require as much volume to resist clinical fracture, which enables a more conservative preparation design.[19] The depth of the restoration is not as significant because adhesive resin systems can be bonded to dentin and enamel and do not require axial wall length to provide frictional retention. In addition, these resin systems have a low elastic modulus for absorbing occlusal stress. Therefore, the properties of dentin are not required. Furthermore, these conservative considerations can be applied to every aspect of restorative dentistry, including the restoration of hard and soft tissue. Restorative procedures including connective tissue grafting, alveolar ridge augmentation, and placement of implants can provide conservative methods to preserve intraoral structures. These conservative treatment avenues not only preserve but also improve the longevity and esthetics of the natural dentition. The third clinical objective of contemporary restorative dentistry is to perpetuate the longevity of the tooth and restoration by increasing the interval of time between replacement restoration.

FACTORS TO CONSIDER FOR TOOTH PREPARATION

a) Thickness or translucency in the gingival area.
b) Soft-tissue health
c) Positioning the gingival margin for esthetics.

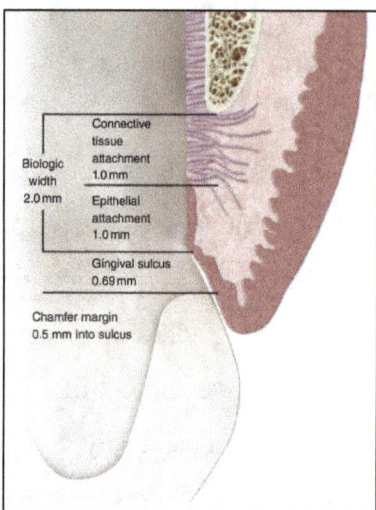

FIGURE 7.1: When preparing a crown margin sub-gingivally, it is important to be aware of the tooth's sulcular depth and to avoid invasion of the biological width. This figure illustrates the structures to consider in this histologic dimension.

TOOTH REDUCTION FOR THE ALL-CERAMIC CROWN

An ideal tooth preparation for the all-ceramic crown is a balanced uniform reduction of tooth structure. Porcelain is strong in compression but quite weak in terms of tensile strength, the full shoulder margin is always used in anterior restorations. Its width can vary from 0.5 to 1.0mm and at times even to 1.5mm. The shoulder is extended halfway or 0.5mm (whichever is greater) into the gingival crevice at a slight apical angle (5°) from the long axis of the tooth. The incisal clearance should be 1.5–2.0mm, with the flat surface at right angles to the surface forces of the occluding teeth.[20] The labial, mesial, distal, and lingual reduction should flow evenly and uniformly about the tooth to a depth of approximately 1mm. Any sharp corners or angles must be rounded. The gingival margin should follow the cementoenamel line smoothly around the tooth.[21]

STEP-BY-STEP TECHNIQUE FOR THE ALL-CERAMIC CROWN

1. **Esthetic depth cut:** A key to the technique is the measured reduction of the horizontal and vertical aspects to a predictable depth. This is accomplished in two steps:

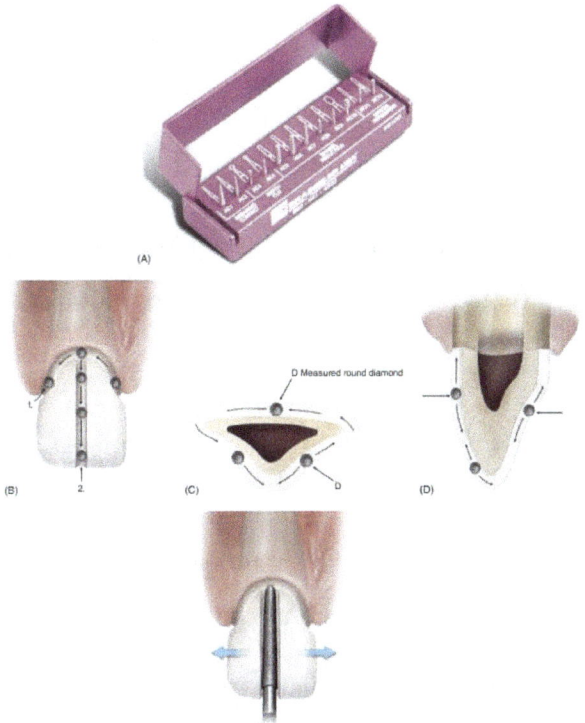

FIGURE 7.2: (A–E) Proper tooth preparation with uniform reduction and rounded internal line angles for an all-ceramic crown using a 12-diamond kit (BrasselerUSA K0100)

(i) **Horizontal depth cut:** Using a premeasured 1.0– 1.5 mm round or AC3 or AC4 (Brasseler USA) diamond bur.

For lower anterior teeth and where significant gingival recession is present, a pre-measured 1.0 mm round diamond should be used (AC4, Brasseler USA).

(ii) **Vertical depth cut:** Therefore, if you are increasing the depth of the buccal and/or lingual walls to 1.5mm, then switch to the AC3 diamond bur, which is 1.5mm in thickness.

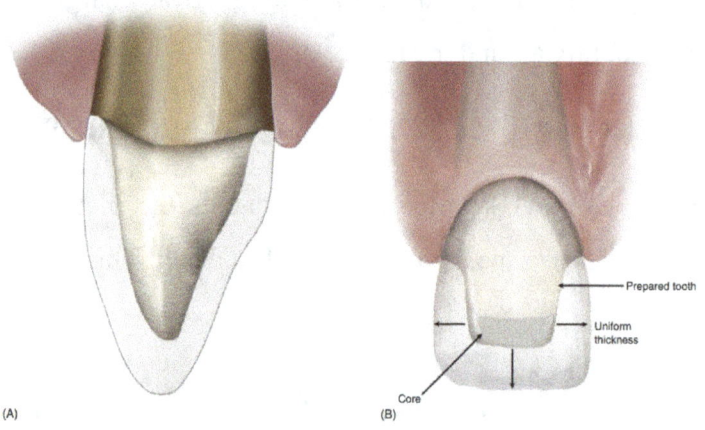

FIGURE 7.3: (A, B) The principles of uniform thickness for a typical all-porcelain crown.

iii) **Bulk enamel removal:** For the esthetic depth cuts use a very coarse round-end tapered diamond bur to remove both enamel and dentin (AC5 or AC7, Brasseler USA). For mandibular anterior teeth use the smaller AC7 for bulk reduction. This diamond will also be useful to reduce interproximal contacts, in extremely small or narrow teeth, use the AC9 diamond.

iv) **Incisal/occlusal clearance:** Using the same round-end tapered diamond bur, reduce the incisal surface by approximately 1.5mm to obtain proper clearance.

v) **Lingual reduction:** A very coarse football-shaped diamond (AC10, Brasseler USA) is used to uniformly reduce the contours of the lingual surface of anterior teeth.

The AC10 (Brasseler USA) is ideal to reduce the occlusal aspect of posterior teeth as well.

Either a plastic or rubber thickness gauge can be used to make certain that your predetermined sufficient space is created.

Also, if you are using a CAD/CAM intraoral scanner (Itero, Align) for your impression taking, the bite registration scan will easily show you if there is sufficient space. If not, you will be prompted to reduce more in those areas, so your restoration can be fabricated with sufficient thickness to avoid a potential fracture.

Margin refinement Preparation and refining of the shoulder margin are easily accomplished with beveled-end cutting diamond (AC11 and AC12, Brasseler USA) shapes.

vi) **Preparation finish**: The preparation is finished to a smoother surface using the same size but round-end tapered diamond used to make the original enamel reduction margin but with medium diamond grit (AC6 or AC8, Brasseler USA).

PORCELAIN-FUSED-TO-METAL RESTORATION

Since its introduction into dentistry in the early 1950s, the ceramo-metal crown gained popularity up until the new millennium, when the all-ceramic crowns achieved more popularity. However, the ceramo-metal crown continues to be a popular prosthetic choice for crowns primarily because it combines the strength and adaptability of metal with the esthetic beauty and durability of porcelain.

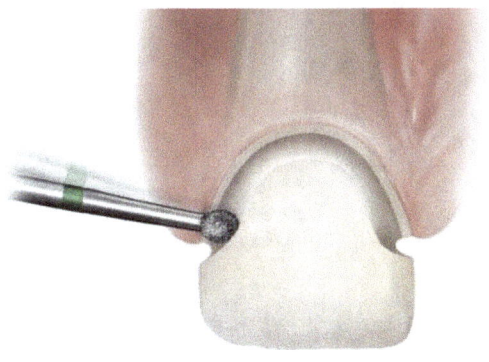
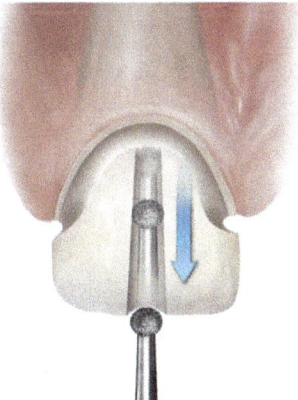

FIGURE 7.4: Esthetic depth determination is both easily and quickly done using premeasured round diamond stones. A round diamond (Brasseler AC4) is used to create horizontal depth cuts at the gingival level, completely around the labial and lingual surfaces.

Vertical depth cut. The depth cut is continued utilizing the same bur through the inciso-gingival dimension. This depth may vary depending on the final desired buccolingual dimension.

TOOTH PREPARATIONS

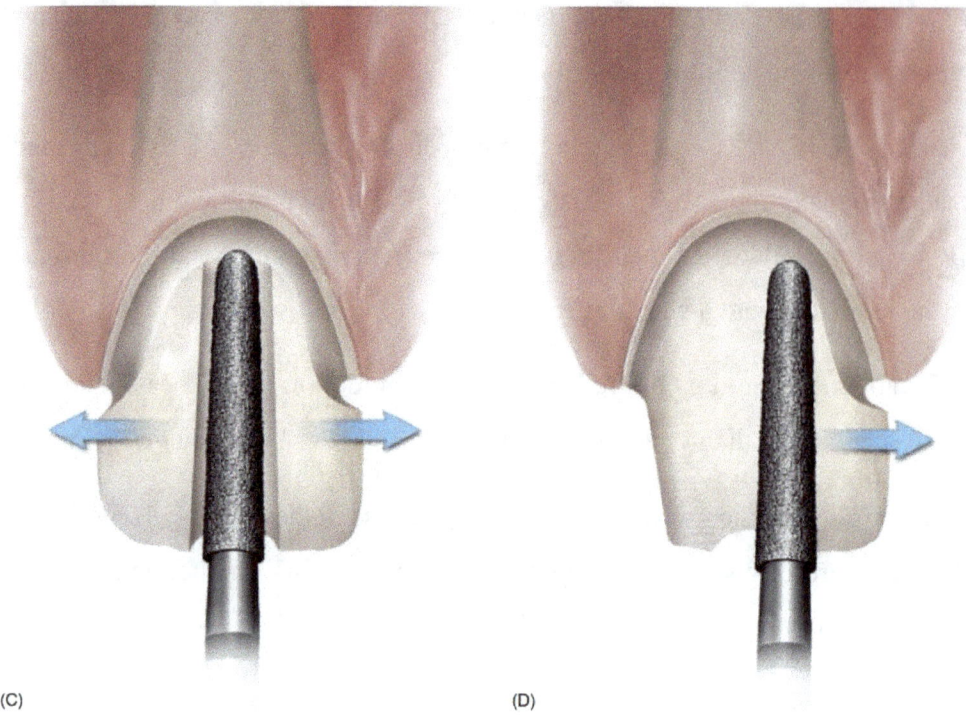

(C)   (D)

FIGURE 7.4: (C, D) Bulk enamel removal. Following the vertical depth cut, an extra-coarse round-end tapered diamond (Brasseler AC5 or AC7) is utilized to remove enamel and dentin to the desired depth.

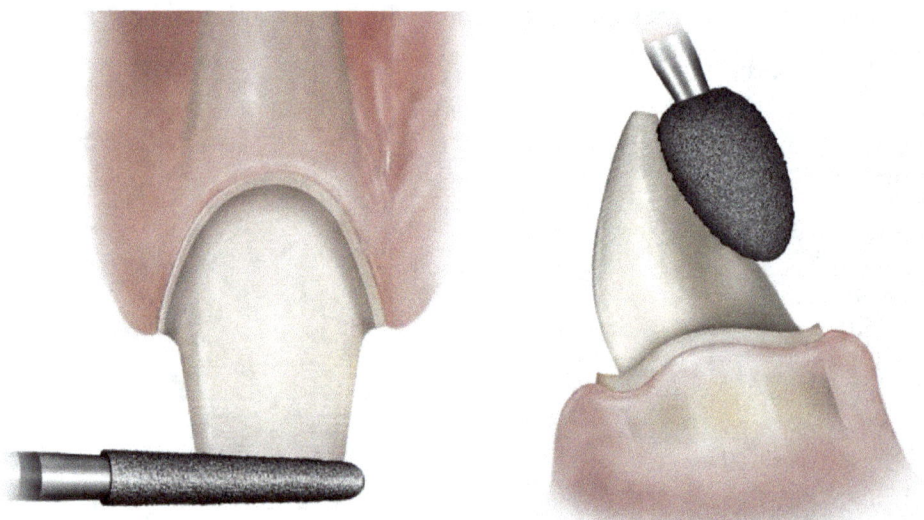

FIGURE 7.5: Incisal clearance. Using the same round-end tapered diamond, incisal reduction is completed using the same round-end diamond (AC5, Brasseler USA) to achieve proper clearance with the opposing dentition. Lingual reduction. The AC10 diamond (Brasseler) is used to obtain proper lingual reduction and contours.

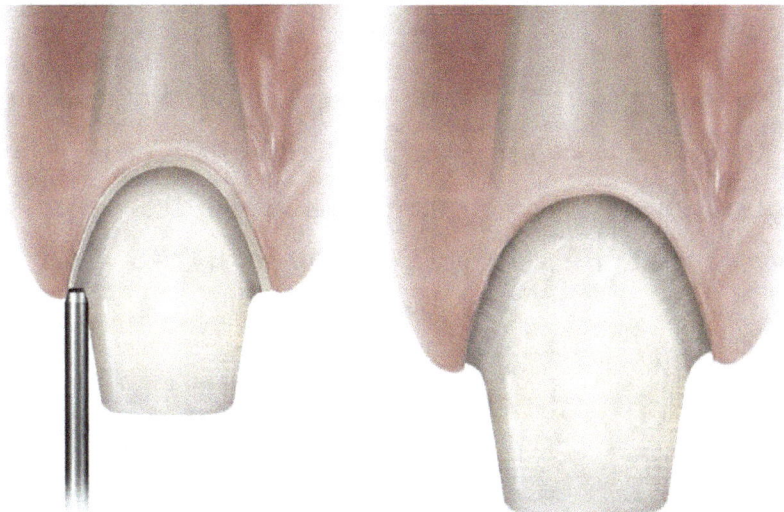

FIGURE 7.6: Margin refinement. Preparation and refining of the margin are done with the beveled end-cutting diamond (Brasseler AC11 or AC12). The beveled-end shape helps to prevent internal line angle undercuts as well as avoid gingival abrasion.[22-29]

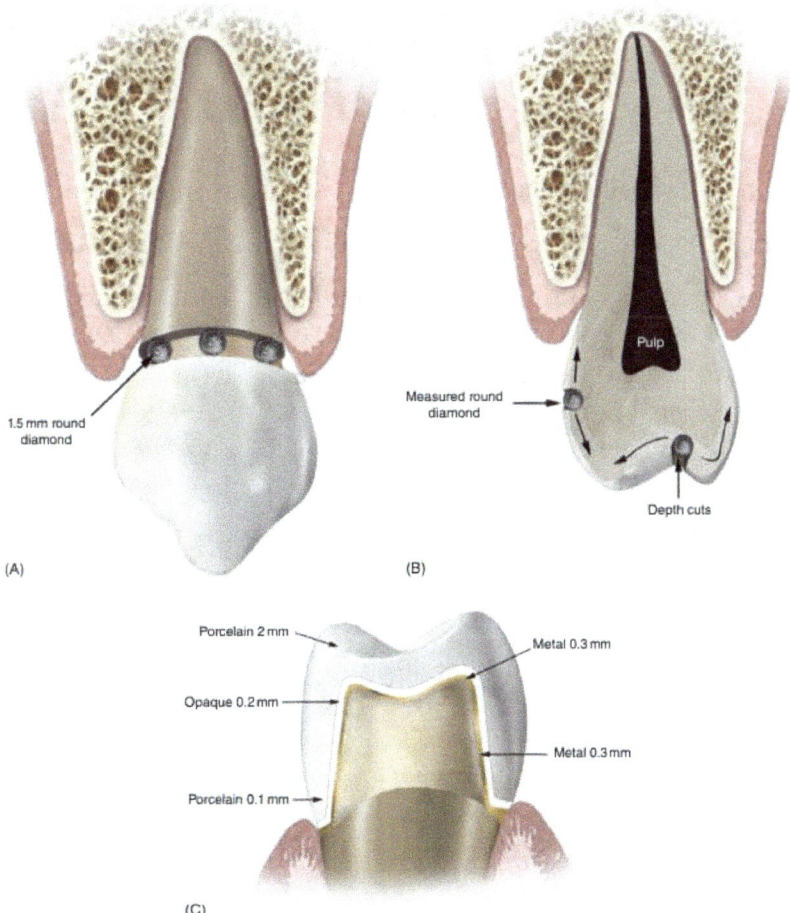

FIGURE 7.7: (A–C) As with the anterior teeth, esthetic depth determination is both easily and quickly done using premeasured round diamond stones.

Types of margins

The determination and preparation of the cervical margin is one of the most important and esthetically critical steps in tooth preparation. As **Berman** states, to provide adequate room for the terminal margin of the crown, the portion of the tooth in the sulcus must be adequately exposed either by retraction, laser, or electrosurgery.[27]

The shoulder [10, 32]

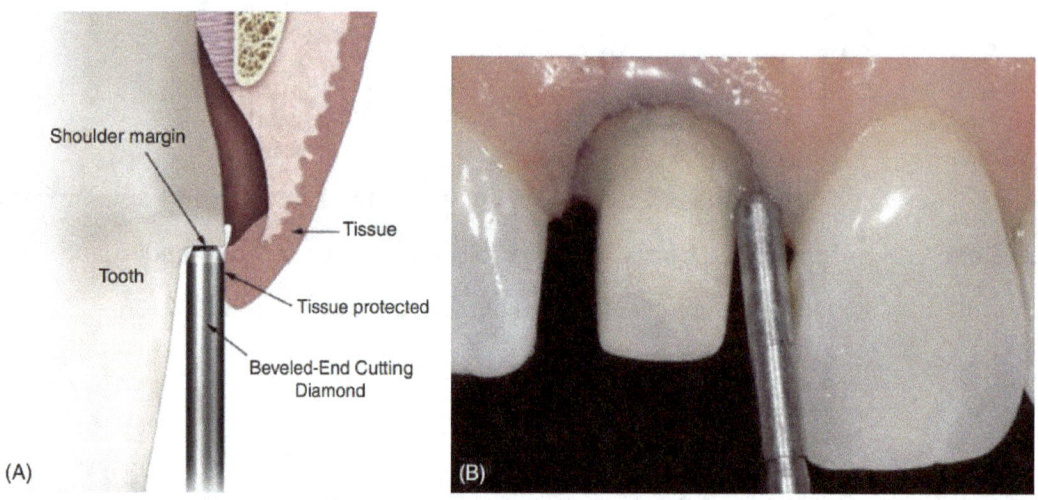

FIGURE 7.8: (A, B) This illustration and clinical example show appropriate use of the beveled-end cutting diamond (Brasseler AC11 and AC12) to finish subgingival margins while protecting the gingival tissue. Note the use of gingival retraction in (B).

Classification of tooth preparation for anterior veneers

The following is based on the present evidence-based literature.[28-36]

Class 0: No preparation.

Class 1: Window preparation (window). Veneer ends below the incisal edge.

Class 2: Feather-edged preparation technique (feather). Veneer extends to the incisal edge; there is no reduction of the incisal edge.

Class 3: Bevel preparation (bevel/small butt joint). Buccopalatal bevel; there is a reduction of the incisal edge.

Class 4: Overlapping preparation of incisal edges (incisal overlap). Reduction of the incisal edge and palatal extension of the preparation.

Class 5: Butt joint preparation. Incisal reduction of ≥2mm, 90° lingual marginal finish. Interproximal preparation includes the contact areas.

Class 6: Full veneer preparation (complete veneer, ¾ veneer). Interproximal and palatal preparation extension, including palatal deep chamfer or rounded shoulder preparation. Variable defect-oriented preparation; a hybrid between the veneer and all-ceramic crown.[21,27]

The classic veneer preparation technique

The Goldstein veneer preparation kit (LVS; Brasseler USA) provides a rapid method of measured reduction for porcelain veneers. First, the clinician must decide on the required amount of reduction, using the considerations given previously.

In most instances, the needed reduction will be 0.5mm, obtained by using the LVS-1. Small teeth such as the mandibular incisors where the thickness of enamel is considerably less may only require a 0.3mm reduction and you would use LVS-2.

The remaining enamel is then reduced to the depth of these initial cuts, using a coarse diamond (LVS-3 or -4).

At the marginal areas, however, it is desirable to use a finer-grit diamond for a definitive polished finish line to enhance the seal at the periphery, the special two-grit LVS-3 or -4 is an ideal instrument to accomplish these tasks.

If the margin is planned to be placed subgingivally, it is best to begin by displacing the tissue with a retraction cord saturated with a hemostatic agent.

The final margin using the LVS-3.

THE NOVEL EXTENDED VENEER PREPARATION TECHNIQUE

Both, the overlapping incisal edge preparation (modified overlap design; **Stappert** 1999) and the full veneer preparation design (**Stappert** 1999) include the proximal tooth surfaces but differ in palatal extension. The extent of tooth structure defect and the functional and esthetic objectives of the therapy determine the choice of preparation design. The extended veneer preparation kits combine classic crown burs with veneer burs. They are performed initially with rough diamond burs (80 μm).

TOOTH PREPARATIONS

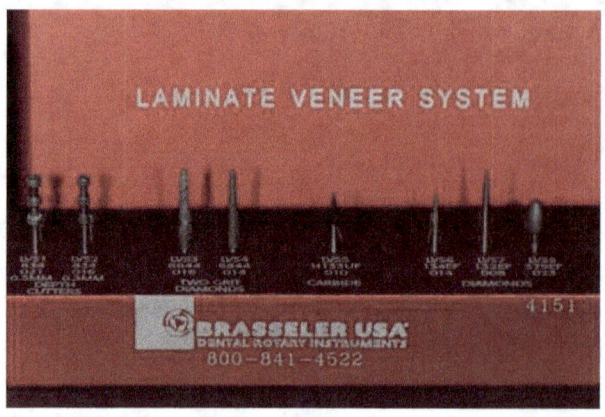

FIGURE 7.9: This veneer system (Brasseler USA) includes four burs to prepare the tooth and four to finish the veneer.

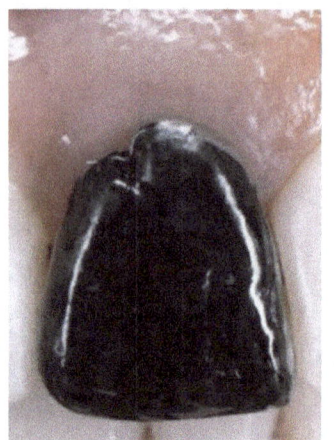 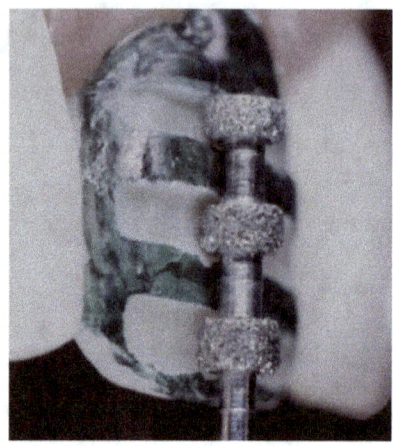 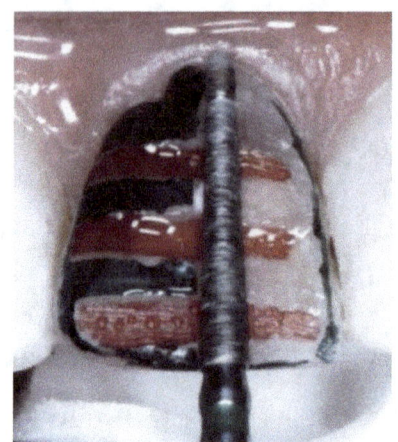

FIGURE 7.10: The discolored incisor is painted green to help guide the depth cuts. The special three-tier extra-coarse diamond depth cutter (Brasseler USA) in 0.5mm (LVS-1) and 0.3mm (LVS-2) thicknesses and is so efficient that usually one sweep across the labial surface completes the depth cut.

#837KR.314.012, #878.204.012; (Brasseler USA) followed by finer shape-congruent diamond burs (30–40 μm) #8837KR.314.012, #8878.204.012; (Brasseler USA) for the finishing procedure.

The extent of labial and incisal reduction is pre-determined for both preparation forms by using a silicone key based on an esthetic functional wax-up. The labial surface is axially reduced by 0.3–0.5mm. Cervically, a shallow chamfer (0.5mm) is prepared epi-gingival. The proximal reduction is 0.5–0.7mm. The incisal edge is shortened by a minimum of 0.5–1.5mm for both preparation forms using #837KR.314.012; (Brasseler USA), depending on the defect size.

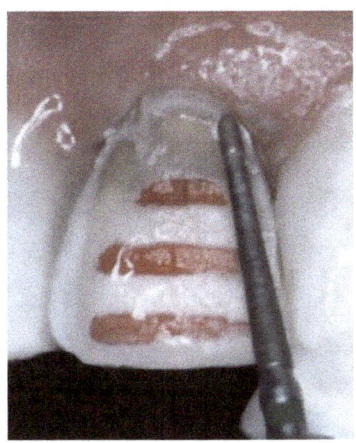 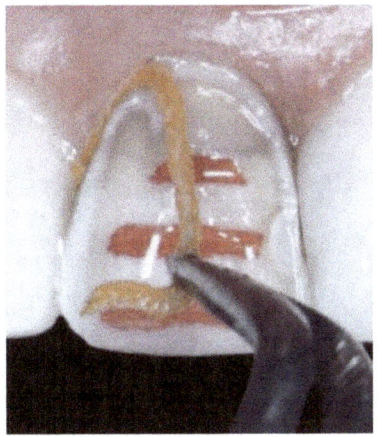 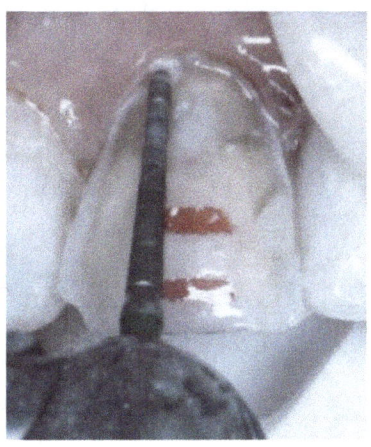

FIGURE 7.11: The tip of the two-grit diamond LVS-3 or -4 (Brasseler USA) has a fine grit for marginal finishing. Note how close the preparation was finished to the base of the depth cut as shown by the remaining illustrative red markings.

Gingival displacement cord is carefully removed after remaining in the sulcus for approximately 10min.

With the tissue displaced, the gingival margin can now be placed just into the gingival sulcus

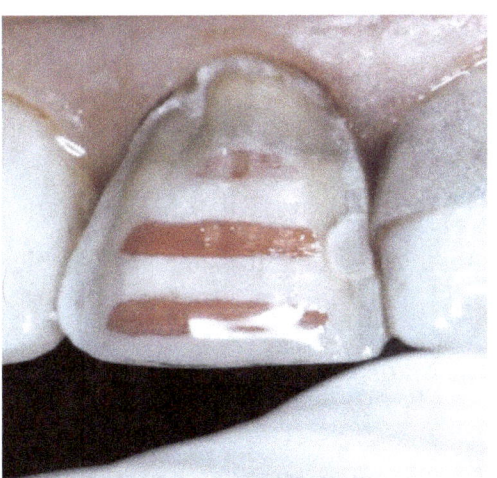 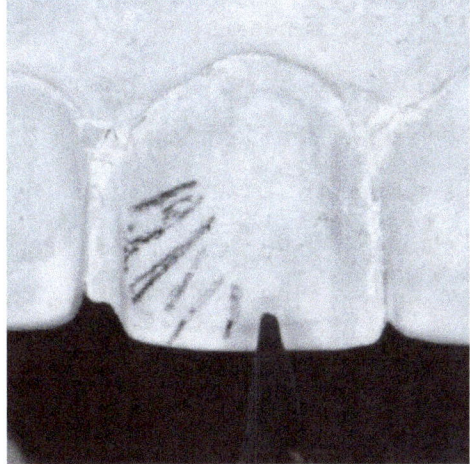

FIGURE 7.12: When using the foil technique for veneer construction (see the section on Foil versus refractory die), slight separation between the teeth is obtained by using diamond strips. The proximal surfaces can then be finished with a sandpaper strip.

An initial impression is made of the completed preparations and poured in quick-set plaster or stone to carefully analyze each tooth. Here the distal-labial aspect appears to need slightly more reduction.

REFERENCES

1. **Osborne JW, Summitt JB.** Extension for prevention: Is it relevant today? Am J Dent 1998; 11:189-196.
2. **Webb MH.** Restoration of contour and prevention of extension of decay. Brit J Dent Sci 1881; 24:1117-1124.
3. **Black GV.** Management of enamel margins. Dent Cosmos 1891; 33:85—100.
4. **Simonsen RJ.** Conservation of tooth structure in restorative dentistry. Quintessence Int 1985; 16:15-24.
5. **Black GV.** A Work on Operative Dentistry, vol 1. Chicago: Medico-dental, 1917.
6. **Mount GJ, Hume WR.** A new cavity classification. Aust Dent J 1998; 43:153-159.
7.
7. **Welk DA, Laswell HR.** The rationale for designing cavity preparations in light of current knowledge and technology. Dent Clin North Am 1976; 20:231-239. 8.
8. **Mount GJ, Ngo H.** Minimal intervention: Early lesions. Quintessence Int 2000;31:535-546.
9. **White JM, Eakle WS.** Rationale and treatment approach in minimally invasive dentistry. J Am Dent Assoc 2000;131 suppl:13S-19S.
10. **Dawson AS, Makinson OF.** Dental treatment and dental health. Part 2. An alternative philosophy and some new treatment modalities in operative dentistry. Aust Dent J 1992; 37:205-210.
11. **Charland R, Prevost A** Conservative restoration with composite resins [in French]. J Dent Que 1990; 27:361-364.
12. **Laswell HR, Welk DA.** The rationale for designing cavity preparations. Dent Clin North Am 1985; 29:241-249.
13. **Peters MC, McLean ME.** Minimally invasive operative care. I. Minimal intervention and concepts for minimally invasive cavity preparations. J Adhes Dent 2001; 3:7—16.
14. **Heinrich-Weltzien R, Kuhnisch J, van der Veen M, de Josselin de Jong E, Stosser L.** Quantitative light-induced fluorescence (QLF)—A potential method for the dental practitioner. Quintessence Int 2003;34:181-188.
15. **Mount GJ, Hume WR.** Preservation and Restoration of Tooth Structure. London: Mosby, 1998.

16. **Mount GJ, Ngo H.** Minimal intervention: Advanced lesions. Quintessence Int 2000; 31:621— 629.

17. **Hosoda H, Fukuyama T.** A tooth substance saving restorative technique. Int Dent J 1984; 34:1-12.

18. **Lutz F.** State of the art of tooth-colored restoratives. Oper Dent 1996; 21:237-248.

19. **Leinfelder KF.** A conservative approach to placing posterior composite resin restorations. J Am Dent Assoc 1996; 127:743-748.

20. **Johnston JF, Mumford G, Dykema RW.** Modern Practice in Dental Ceramics. Philadelphia, PA: W.B. Saunders; 1967.

21. **Mumford G, Ridge A.** Dental porcelain. Dent Clin North Am 1971; 15:33–42.

22. **Straussberg G, Katz G, Kuwota M.** Design of gold supporting structures for fused porcelain restorations. J Prosthet Dent 1966; 16:928–936.

23. **Huttner G.** Follow-up study of crowns and abutments with regard to the crown edge and the marginal periodontium. Dtsch Zahnärztl Z 1971; 26:724–729 [in German].

24. **Brecker SC.** Procedures to improve esthetics in restorative dentistry. J N Carolina Dent Soc 1957; 41:33–36.

25. **Tergis MJ.** The proper geometry of preparation and case design in porcelain-on-gold restorations. J Acad Gen Dent 1971; 19:15–17.

26. **Stein RS.** A dentist and a dental technologist analyze current ceramo-metal procedures. Dent Clin N Am 1977; 4:729–749.

27. **Berman MH.** Cutting efficiency in complete coverage preparation. J Am Dent Assoc 1969; 79:1160–1167.

28. **Stappert CF, Ozden U, Gerds T, Strub JR.** Longevity and failure load of ceramic veneers with different preparation designs after exposure to masticatory simulation. J Prosthet Dent 2005; 94:132–139.

29. **Guess PC, Stappert CF.** Midterm results of a 5-year prospective clinical investigation of extended ceramic veneers. Dent Mater 2008;24(6):804–813.

30. **Stappert CF, Ozden U, Att W, et al.** Marginal accuracy of press-ceramic veneers influenced by preparation design and fatigue. Am J Dent 2007; 20:380–384. 26.

31. **Stappert CF, Stathopoulou N, Gerds T, Strub JR.** Survival rate and fracture strength of maxillary incisors, restored with different kinds of full veneers. J Oral Rehabil 2005; 32:266–272.

32. **Belser UC, Magne P, Magne M.** Ceramic laminate veneers: continuous evolution of indications. J Esthet Dent 1997; 9:197–207.

33. **Walls AW, Steele JG, Wassell RW.** Crowns and other extra-coronal restorations: porcelain laminate veneers. Br Dent J 2002; 193:73– 76, 79–82. 61.

34. **Calamia JR.** Etched porcelain facial veneers: a new treatment modality based on scientific and clinical evidence. NY J Dent 1983; 53:255–259. 62.

35. **Crispin BJ.** Expanding the application of facial ceramic veneers. J Calif Dent Assoc 1993; 21:43–46, 48–49, 52–44. 63.

36. **el-Sherif M, Jacobi R.** The ceramic reverse three-quarter crown for anterior teeth: preparation design. J Prosthet Dent 1989; 61:4–6

CHAPTER-8
CERAMICS

Ceramics is derived from the Greek word Keramos, which was the ancient art of fabricating pottery. This word may have originated from a Sanskrit term meaning burnt earth because the main constituents were clays excavated from the earth, which were heated to form pottery.[1-2] Although the methods of acquiring, purifying, and fabricating these raw materials into ceramic objects have significantly changed, some of the basic materials and techniques are still the same.

Traditional ceramics uses clay as one of its primary components, in combination with other metal oxides including feldspar (K;0Al2O3 6SiO2), alumina (Al2O3), potash (K2O), and soda (Na2O). Ceramic objects are still fabricated by pulverizing these raw materials into fine particles and powders and adding water to help keep the particles together during sculpting and shaping. The "green"(unbaked) object is dried and placed into an oven (kiln) and heated to a specified temperature that allows the individual particles to coalesce into a solid mass. The process of coalescence of the particles is called sintering, and it usually results in shrinkage and strengthening of the solid mass. These traditional ceramics include stoneware (tile), earthenware (pottery), porcelain (tableware and china), electrical insulators, bricks, and sanitary ware (sinks and toilets).[3]

PROPERTIES OF CERAMIC MATERIAL

Ceramic materials have been part of the dental armamentarium for a considerable length of time. Applications for this highly inert material are quite extensive.

Some of these include porcelain jackets, porcelain fused to metal, inlays/ onlays, core materials, and veneers.[1-4] Their most important properties include color stability, relative insolubility in the oral cavity, and excellent wear resistance. While the compressive strength of porcelain is quite high, ductility and impact strength are relatively low. Consequently, the potential for application is restricted. The introduction of the porcelain-fused-to-metal (PFM) concept made it possible to use porcelain as a partial denture material for both anterior and posterior teeth. The objection to the presence of metal from an esthetic point of view was later overcome by the introduction of alumina and zirconium substrates. The incorporation of both metals and ceramic substrates also increased the fracture resistance of the restoration. One of the more interesting substrates is the machined zirconia ceramic agent. Not only does it provide a metal-free restoration, but it also possesses the potential for arresting the propagation of cracks or fracture lines. Unique to zirconium dioxide, the region immediately at the head of the advancing crack is put in a state of compression. This phenomenon is caused by a transition from one crystalline structure to another. Because the volume of the second structure is different from that of the first, a state of compression is generated, thereby arresting crack advancement. Several mechanical properties are significant in evaluating the clinical performance of ceramic materials. These mechanical properties include flexural strength, fracture toughness, and modulus of elasticity.

CLASSIFICATION OF ALL-CERAMIC SYSTEMS

The following general types of all-ceramic systems are currently available.

- Conventional feldspathic ceramic systems
- Machinable ceramic systems
- Pressable ceramic systems
- Infiltrated ceramic systems

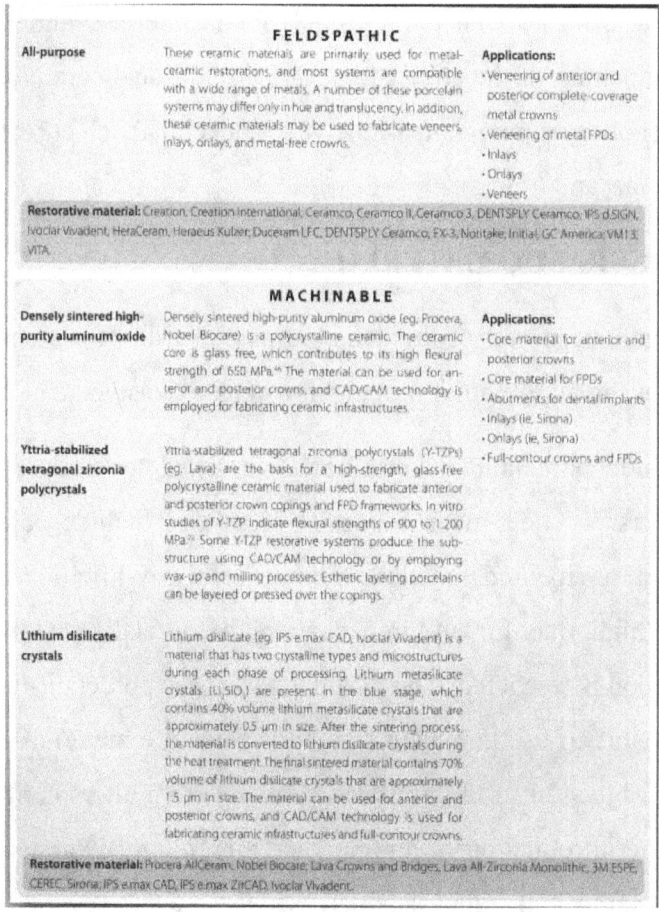

FIGURE 8.1: CLASSIFICATION AND RESTORATIVE APPLICATION OF ALL-CERAMIC SYSTEMS

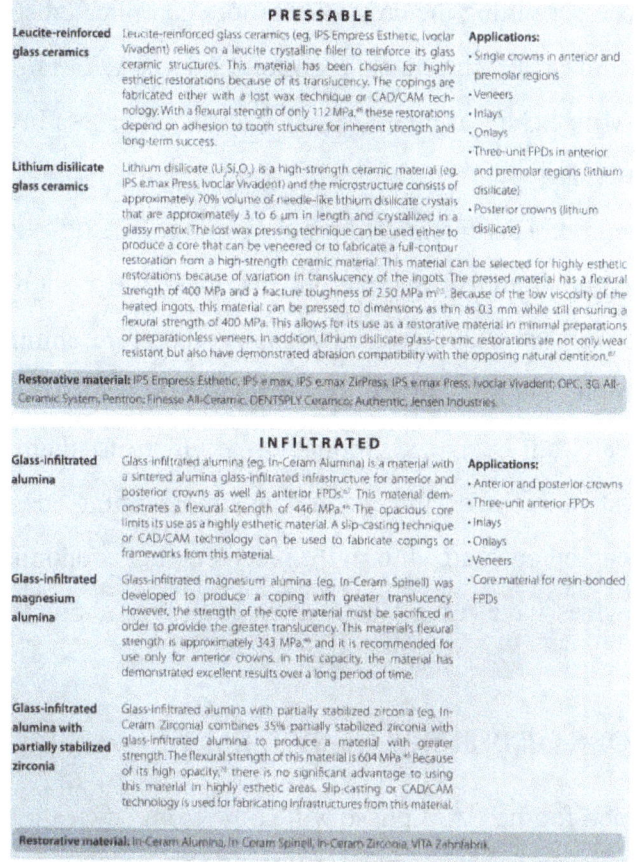

FIGURE 8.2: CONTINUED CLASSIFICATION AND RESTORATIVE APPLICATION OF ALL-CERAMIC SYSTEMS

METHODS FOR FABRICATION OF A ZIRCONIA SINGLE-COPING OR FPD FRAMEWORK

There are two different methods for the fabrication of a zirconia single-coping or FPD framework:

1) Manually controlled system or MAD/MAM method: Referred to as copy milling, this method uses exact mechanical-tactile model surveying and analogous milling4 to ensure precision in transfer accuracy. First, a coping or framework pattern is manually fabricated in composite or acrylic, after which the pattern is placed into a pantographic machine. While the copying arm of the machine traces the pattern, the cutting arm mills a pre-sintered zirconia block with a carbide cutter. Because of shrinkage that will occur during the sintering step, the milled restoration is 20% to 25% larger than the final sintered framework. Although it requires more fabrication time than CAD/CAM scanning systems, this manual method of milling allows the dental technician to alter deficiencies in the die that CAD/CAM systems could not

correct, therefore permitting the creation of more complicated structures. These types of milling machines (ie, Zirkonzahn, Zirkonzahn USA; Ceramill, Amann Girrbach Gmbh; TiZan Mill, Schutz Dental Group) also re- quire less investment than typical CAD/CAM systems.

2) CAD/CAM method: This method of single-coping and FPD framework fabrication involves the manipulation of a three-dimensional (3D) design on the computer. A virtual die and framework are created digitally, therefore eliminating the need for a wax-up. A computer-controlled milling machine104 with automated production is used to fabricate an oversized framework, which is then fully sintered. The CAD/CAM system includes three components: scanning, designing, and milling. Each of these can be outsourced to milling centers, but economical desktop scanning and milling devices have recently allowed the usage of this technology in smaller laboratories.

SCANNING METHODS OF DIFFERENT SYSTEMS

The information obtained for the CAM phase will come from either the CAD phase (ie, Lava Crowns and Bridges, Zirkonzahn, KaVo EVEREST ZS-Blanks) or a scan of a wax/composite coping/framework (ie, Cercon). In each system, a representation of the prepared teeth (ie, CAD/CAM) or wax-up of a coping or framework (i.e., CAM only) must first be acquired and digitized onto the computer monitor. Different systems use different scanning methods. These types of scanning methods include optical cameras, contact digitization (ie, mechanical scanner), and white or colored light or laser projection.[5,6]

One chairside system (ie, CEREC 3D System, Sirona) uses an intraoral optical camera to produce a digital image of the prepared tooth and the adjacent teeth. A charge-coupled device (CCD) camera is employed in another system (ie, KaVo EVEREST) to produce a digital 3D model generated by computing, recording, and merging dense point clouds from 15 different angles and positions.[5]

Another system (i.e., Procera) reads the surface of a stone master die of the prepared tooth using a sphere or scanning stylus that is in contact with the stone surface. This information is electronically sent to one of the two milling centers for the fabrication of the coping or framework. One particular system (i.e., Lava Chairside Oral Scanner C.O.S.) uses a triangulated, white-light optical system to digitize the master model. With this system, not only are the tooth preparations digitized, but also full anatomical contours can be developed from an internal library or scanned in manually.

CAD software

Since the advent of CAD/CAM technology, most systems have been closed architecture (ie, the CAD software information was specific to its CAM unit), which only permits the system to communicate with equipment from one manufacturer. The disadvantage of a closed system architecture is that a laboratory is restricted and limited to whatever products the manufacturer's CAM system provides. However, recently more companies are opening their interfaces for industrial standard formats,[7] and thus by using the standard template library (STL) open file format, data can be sent to any CAM system that accepts STL. This al- lows dental laboratories to choose different material suppliers and not be restricted to one manufacturer's technology. In general, CAD software allows the operator to design the appropriate dental prosthesis step by step. The software program mimics the same steps (i.e., margin selection, block-out of any undercuts, placement of a die spacer for a cement layer) that the dental technician would follow to fabricate a single metal coping or an FPD framework. In a clinical situation with multiple abutments, the path of insertion can be analyzed, and, if necessary, the abutment can be telescoped to optimize the path of insertion. The data can be sent electronically to a compatible off-site milling center (see Figs 1 to 10). For clinical communication between the clinician and the laboratory technician using digital impression-taking, the ability to use an open, closed, or selectively open architecture is of paramount consideration. The compatibility of the chairside CAD/CAM digital impression system with that of the laboratory CAD/CAM system can provide myriad capabilities for treatment planning, material selection, and restorative applications.

CAD hardware

The production of the zirconia coping or partial denture framework can be completed at the dental laboratory or at an off-site milling center. The actual fabrication can be accomplished using either a subtractive or an additive technique.[8] The more common subtractive technique involves cutting the coping or framework from a solid block. The milling time and type of milling instruments used depend on the type of block (i.e., pre-sintered or fully sintered) employed. The milled size of the coping or framework is also dependent on the amount of shrinkage that will occur during sintering. As aforementioned, sintering is required to achieve maximum strength for pre-sintered blocks. Restorations milled out of sintered monoblock from hard machining will be more accurate in shape with precise dimensions.[9] However, hard machining requires more time, and the machine tools are exposed to heavy wear and therefore can withstand only a short running cycle. Also, there is more risk of introducing microscopic cracks into the ceramic surface. Surface flaws do not occur during soft machining because the shaping is accomplished before the sintering process. Milling white monoblocks requires less time, and there is less wear on the machining tools. However, the accuracy of shape and contour is more crucial with soft-machined restorations because shrinkage must be compensated for and controlled. Both systems have a substantial amount of waste of raw materials. On the zirconia block, there is a barcode that shows the density of the block; this density tells the CAM how oversized to make the framework compensates for the shrinkage that occurs during sintering. The additive technique involves building a coping or partial denture framework by adding material onto a die. When a zirconia material is desired, an oversized metal die must be created prior to the powder application to allow for shrinkage during the sintering process. As the powder is applied to the oversized metal die, it is compacted under isostatic pressure. At this "green" stage, a CAM milling procedure is used to finalize the outside contours of the coping or framework. The coping or framework is removed from the die and sintered at 1,550°C. Selective laser sintering or melting is an alternative fabrication method that is presently producing metal frameworks and is in development for zirconia frameworks. Laser sintering involves the collection of CAD data to create a 3D free-form object. Fusing thin layers of heat-fusing powder with a scanning laser beam creates a single coping or framework. Each scanned layer represents a mathematic cross-section of the CAD model of a single coping or framework. The advantages of this type of fabrication are speed and a lack of wasted raw material.

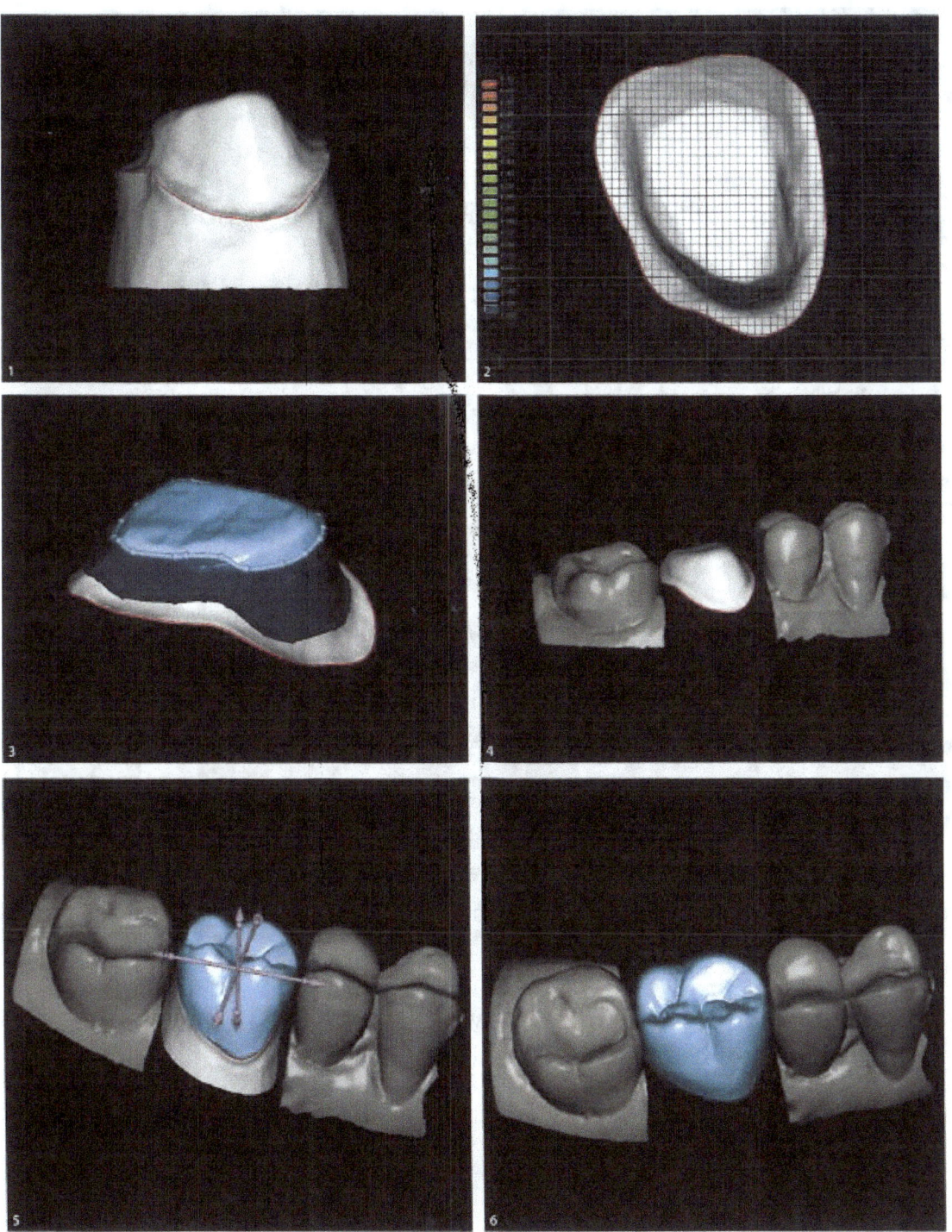

FIGURE 8.3: CAD/CAM SOFTWARE WORKING

CERAMICS

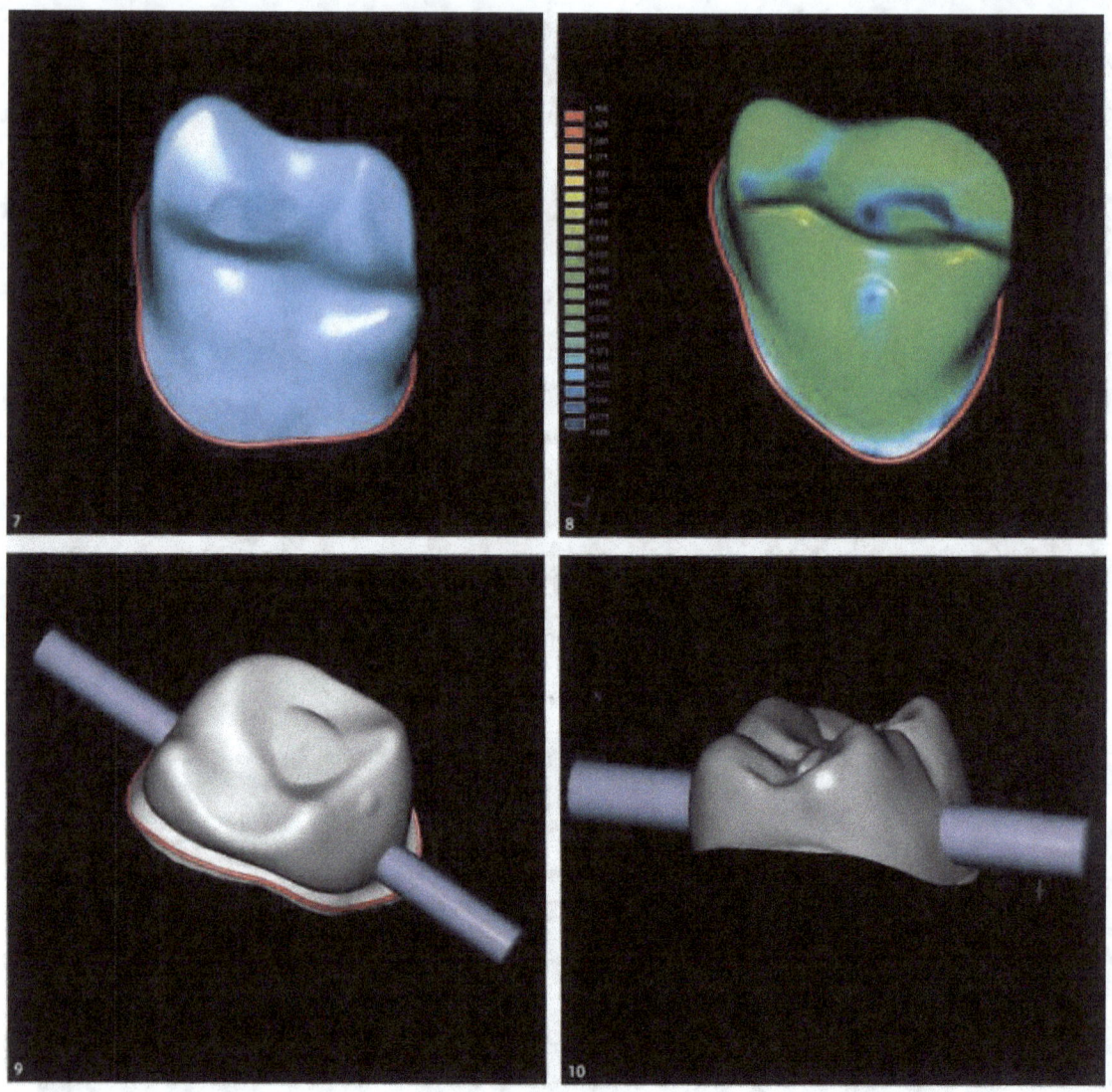

FIGURE 8.3: CAD/CAM SOFTWARE WORK CONTINUED.

REFERENCES

1. **Touati B, Miara P, Nathanson D.** Esthetic Dentistry and Ceramic Restorations. London: Martin Dunitz, 1999.
2. **Frieman S.** Introduction to ceramics and glasses. In: ASM Engineering Materials Handbook, vol 4: Ceramics and Glasses. Philadelphia: ASM International, 1991:1—40.
3. **Kingery WD, Bowen HK, Uhlmann DR.** Introduction to Ceramics, ed 2. New York: John Wiley,1976.
4. **Reichert A, Herkommer D, Muller W.** Copy milling of zirconia.Spectrum Dialogue 2007; 6:40-56.
5. **Liu PR.** A panorama of dental CAD/CAM restorative systems. Compend Contin Educ Dent 2005; 26:507-512. 106.
6. **Witkowski S.** (CAD-)/CAM in dental technology. Quintessence Dent Technol 2005; 28:169-184.
7. **Riqiuer R.** Rapid manufacturing:What will be next.Spectrum Dialogue 2007;6:116-120.
8. **Rekow ED, Silva NR, Coelho PG, Guess P, Thompson VP.** Performance of dental ceramics: Challenges for improvements. J Dent Res 2011; 90:937—952.
9. **Bindl A, Mormann WEI.** The fit of all-ceramic posterior fixed partial denture frameworks in vitro. Int J Periodontics Restorative Dent 2007; 27:567-575.

CHAPTER-9
PROVISIONALIZATION

Restorative treatment concepts of the past regarded the provisional restoration as little more than a space holder to allow the patient to function until the definitive restoration was received from the dental laboratory. The adage "do not make the temporary too nice or the patient will not come back" relied on this philosophy.[1] A temporary restoration of mediocre quality replaced by any significant definitive restoration often pressured or persuaded the patient to accept the definitive restoration.[2] Prosthetic failures arise not only from technical challenges but also from differences in expectations and perceptions of the restoration between the patient, clinician, and technician.[3] The modern restorative treatment concept abandons this original philosophy and utilizes the interim restoration to provide the patient, clinician, and technician with feedback of information while reaffirming the final goals of treatment. The transition in terminology from "temporary" to "treatment" or "interim" restoration reflects the changes in restorative treatment concepts from the past to the present. The interim restoration has become an integral component in the development and management of soft tissue profiles and for the design of the definitive prosthetic restoration.[4-7]

CLINICAL OBJECTIVES OF THE INTERIM RESTORATION

In modern restorative dentistry, interim restoration plays a significant role during the treatment phase for patients who require periodontal therapy and prosthetic dentistry and should fulfill the following clinical objectives[8-23]:

• Protects prepared teeth and the pulp from thermal and chemical influences and exposed dentin from bacterial invasion while reducing dentinal sensitivity.

• Prevents caries and eliminates mechanical defects.

• Supports and stabilizes compromised teeth.

• Provides a guide for tooth reduction.

• Preserves the position, form, and color of the gingiva and maintains the periodontal health while the definitive restoration is being fabricated Serves as a diagnostic tool to determine the appropriate vertical dimension of occlusion, occlusal and incisal planes, incisal length, lip, and tooth position, and facial dimension.

- Maintains tooth position and prevents movement and occlusal changes.

- Stabilizes the maxillomandibular relationship through proper occlusal stability.

- Develops and establishes function, esthetics, and phonetics. Provides physiologic and psychologic comfort to the patient while eliciting patient acceptance of the shape, texture, and color.

- Tests osseointegration of an implant and allows one to develop gingival contours before final rehabilitation.

Assessment of these objectives before developing the final restoration may provide insight into the detection and elimination of potential challenges while evaluating the potential for success of the definitive restorative therapy. These treatment restorations allow proper evaluation of inter-cuspal relation, bruxism, anterior guidance, occlusal vertical dimension, temporomandibular dysfunction symptoms, pulpal vitality, periodontal health, comfort, function, and esthetics.[24] In addition, an evaluation of oral hygiene techniques can provide valuable information for modifying the anatomical design of the final restoration for optimal oral health.

CLINICAL REQUIREMENTS FOR DEVELOPING AN OPTIMAL INTERIM RESTORATION

Unfortunately, many clinicians are still utilizing yesterday's "temporary" restoration concept with today's newer restorative provisional materials and wondering why they have mediocre final results. This "temporary mentality" approach may compromise the placement of high-quality definitive restorations because the time between tooth preparation and the placement of the definitive restoration is insufficient for achieving optimal success.

There are several contributing factors to a well-integrated interim restoration as well as the definitive restoration[25-28]:

- Material stability, strength, and durability (wear resistance)

- Porosity (i.e., nonporous), irritation (i.e., non-irritating), and color stability

- Smooth and highly polished, plaque-resistant surfaces

- Optimal marginal adaptation to tooth preparation ensuring significant restorative seal

- Ideal physiologic contours and embrasures

- Optimal retention during the function

- Ideal occlusal and proximal contacts

- Favorable esthetics

- Comfort during the function

- Cleansability during oral hygiene procedures

- Easy removal and re-cementation

- Optimal gingival adaptation

FABRICATION TECHNIQUES: DIRECT, SEMIDIRECT, AND INDIRECT

The techniques for provisional restoration fabrication vary depending on the specific clinical procedure and restorative objective. Various procedures are available to facilitate short-term biocompatible provisional restorations, including the direct alginate or polyvinyl siloxane over impression technique, indirect matrix technique, block technique, and the laboratory heat-processed technique.[1, 6, 8, 16, 28-31] These techniques use auto-polymerizing acrylic resins, visible light-curing resin,[32, 33] and composites. interim restorations for inlays, crowns, veneers, and fixed partial dentures (FPDs). The direct technique involves using an over-impression developed from an alginate or elastomeric impression material as a template. This direct matrix replicates the exact preoperative tooth structure and soft tissue profiles of the intraoral condition. The impression template is used as a vehicle to transfer the provisional material to the prepared tooth structure.

Another method of the direct technique involves preformed shells to transfer the acrylic resin to the prepared tooth structure.[32] The semidirect technique is based on a combination of in-office laboratory and intraoral procedures. The laboratory procedure involves making a silicone impression matrix of the preoperative stone model or a modified diagnostic wax-up. The custom matrix can be used in the laboratory to transfer the provisional material to the minimally prepared stone model [34,35] or intraorally to the prepared tooth structure. However, it is important to remember that if the provisional is fabricated from the stone model it will need to be relined intraorally with the provisional material after completion of the tooth preparation. Furthermore, each of these techniques can be modified using a cutback technique with the application of tints and modifiers and a final translucent layer of hybrid composite resin. This modification technique can improve color stability, wear resistance, longevity, contour, shape, surface finish, and esthetics.

An alternative semidirect technique that can be applied before veneer preparation is the Aesthetic Pre-evaluative Temporaries (APT).[36, 37] This procedure guides the patient in understanding and accepting the proposed treatment, assuring the expectations of the outcome while directing the preparation and smile design. This technique involves making a clear polyvinyl siloxane matrix of the approved diagnostic wax-up in the laboratory. Individual openings are made on this matrix from the incisal of each modified tooth. The tooth-surface conditioning can vary from spot etching to complete surface etching with an application of adhesive. The clear matrix is applied intraorally, and a flowable composite is injected through each opening onto the unprepared teeth and light cured for 40 seconds from the facial and lingual aspects. These provisional restorations can be fabricated individually or as a group and adhesively bonded. This semidirect technique provides a smile design prototype that can be test driven by the patient and evaluated by the patient, clinician, and technician. In addition, it provides a guide for determining precise dimensions of the tooth preparation in advance, with the potential of conserving tooth structure. This technique can also be applied after veneer preparation for the fabrication of the provisional.

For the fabrication of long-term biologically acceptable multiple provisional restorations, the indirect technique may provide more efficient use of chair time and reduce direct exposure to heat generated by the exothermic polymerization reaction of the auto-polymerizing acrylics. The indirect sandwich technique with a dentin-shaded self-curing acrylic (New Outline dentin, AnaxDent) and characterized through a cutback technique using different tints and modifiers (Kolor + Plus, Kerr/ Sybron) while a translucent acrylic enamel layer (New Outline, High Value or Low Value, AnaxDent) is pressed over the dentin core. These indirect acrylic resin provisionals can be heat processed in a hydro flask for improved color stability, resistance to wear, esthetics, and longevity.[38] However, for optimal functional and esthetic results, an accurate polyvinyl or polyether impression of the final preparations is required, followed by mounting casts with appropriate interocclusal records and custom color selection as required by the laboratory. An initial direct provisional is usually required during the fabrication of the interim laboratory restoration. Although these indirect provisionals can provide optimal material strength, stability, and durability, they require additional laboratory expenses and can be more time-consuming.[29, 39]

CONSIDERATION FACTORS IN CEMENT SELECTION

The selection of an appropriate luting cement for a provisional restoration may appear insignificant. However, improper selection may cause various complications, including leakage; recurrent decay; loss of the provisional restoration; migration of the prepared, adjacent, and opposing dentition; and the potential for fracture of the preparation. For an optimal selection process, the clinician should have knowledge of the following:

• Clinical conditions (e.g., caries index of the patient)

-Preparation design (i.e., degree of mechanical retention)

-Underlying restorative foundation (i.e., core buildup, type of post)

• Mechanical forces (e.g., parafunctional habits)

-Type of provisional restoration (i.e., full- or partial-coverage, single-unit, fixed or partial denture abutment)

- Final restorative material

-Biologic, physical, and handling properties of the luting agent

-Anticipated length of provisional period [40]

Thus, to improve the selection process, the following requisites for selecting the proper provisional cement should be considered:

- Optimal retention during the function
- Favorable esthetics
- Provides ease of removal and cleanup
- Adequate extraoral working time
- Time period for a provisional restoration
- Relining of provisional
- Effect on bond strength

PROVISIONALIZATION

LABORATORY FABRICATION OF A COMPOSITE RESIN FIXED PARTIAL DENTURE

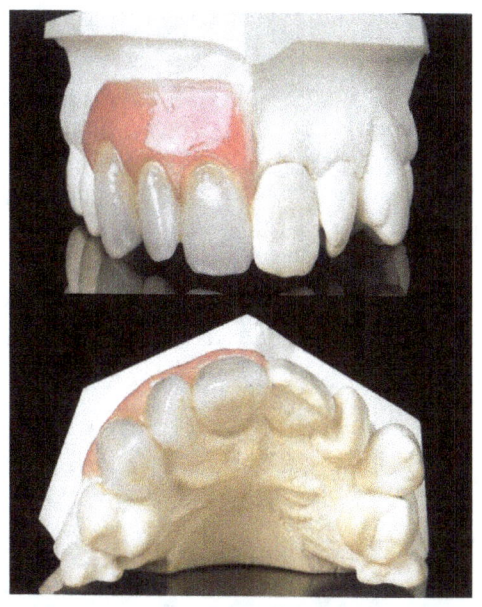

The facial and occlusal views of the completed diagnostic wax-up (Master Diagnostic Model, Valley Dental Arts Laboratory) for an FPD are shown (Figs 1 and 2).

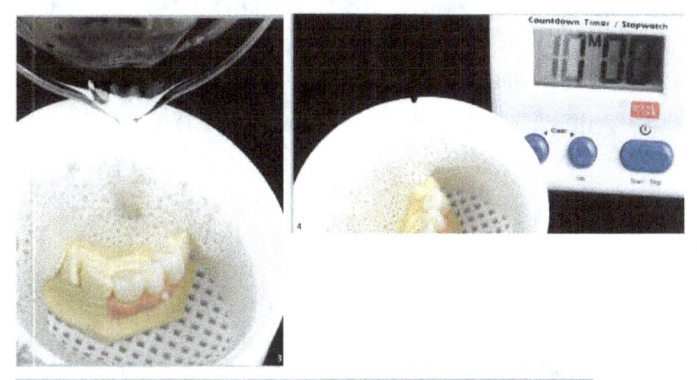

A mixture of soap and water was poured into a container, and the diagnostic wax-up was soaked in this soapy mixture for 10 minutes (Figs 3 and 4).

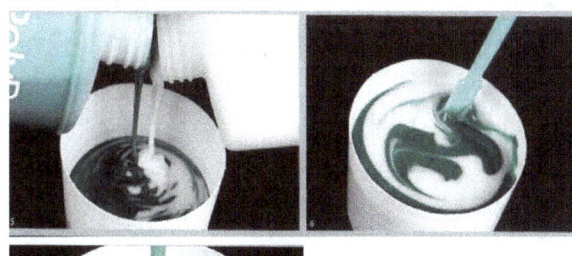

An equal volume of silicone catalyst and base (PolyPour, GC America) was mixed thoroughly into a homogenous liquid (Figs 5 and 6).

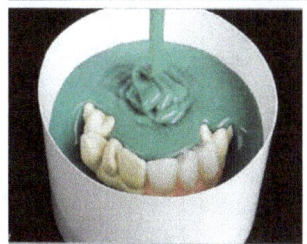

The diagnostic wax-up was duplicated by making a silicone investment (Fig 7).

PROVISIONALIZATION

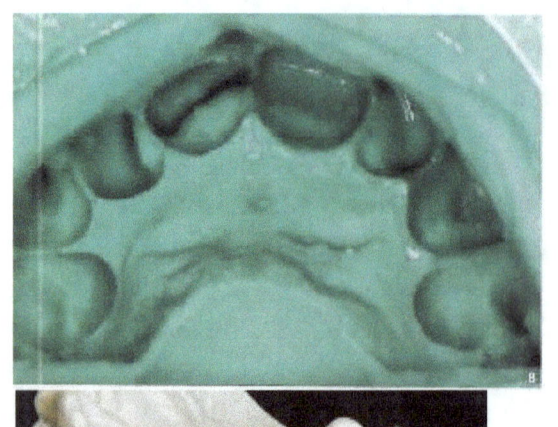

Figure 8 shows the precise silicone impression of the diagnostic wax-up.

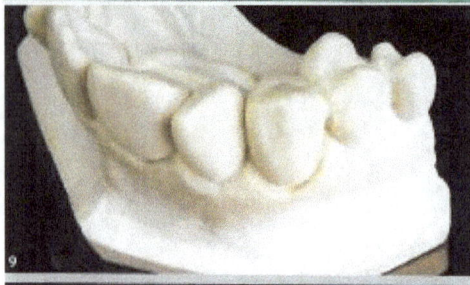

An exact duplicate stone model (GC Fuji Rock ER GC America) was made from the silicone impression (Fig 9).

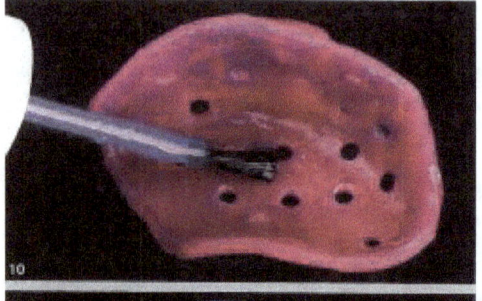

A custom acrylic tray (Palatray XL, Heraeus Kulzer) was fabricated from the stone model, and a universal adhesive was applied (Universal Adhesive, Heraeus Kulzer) (Fig 10).

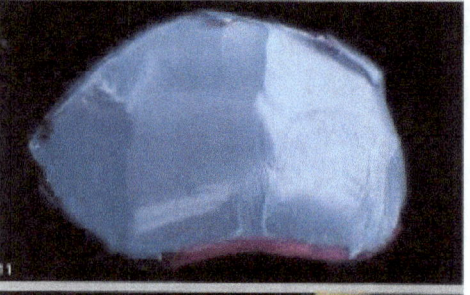

A heavy-body polyvinyl impression material was loaded into the custom tray, and a light-body polyvinyl impression material was injected around the cervical region of the teeth on the model (Figs 11 and 12).

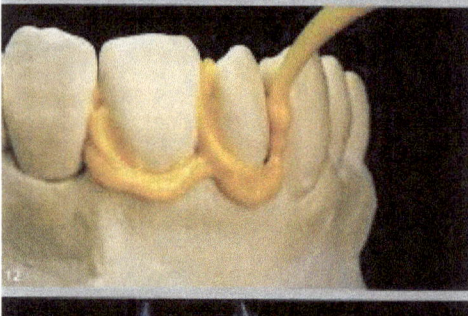

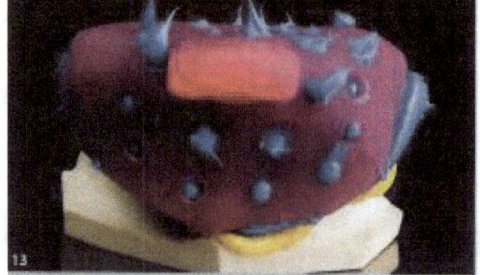

The tray was precisely positioned onto the stone model and allowed to set for 4 to 6 minutes (Fig 13)

PROVISIONALIZATION

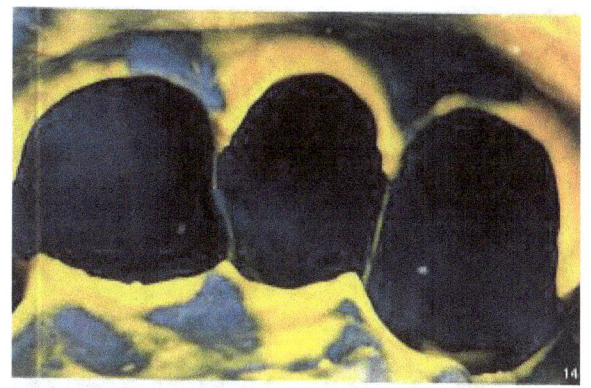

The polyvinyl impression of the duplicate model can be used as a vehicle transfer for the bis-acryl resin (Fig 14).

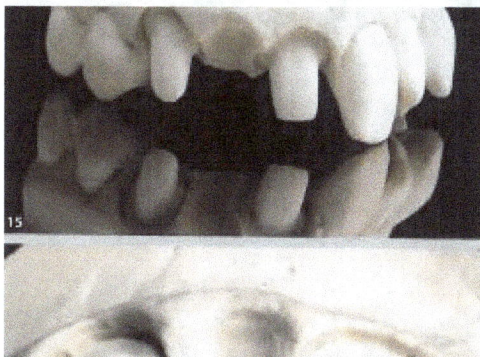

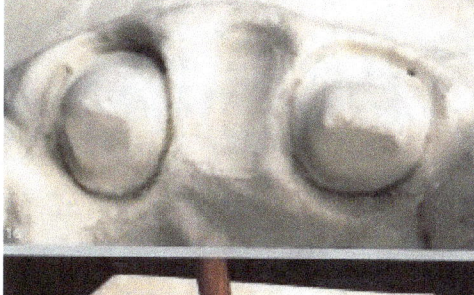

Figures 15 and 16 show the facial and occlusal views of the preparation. y model made from either an intraoral impression of preparations or an impression of laboratory preparations made on a duplicate stone model.

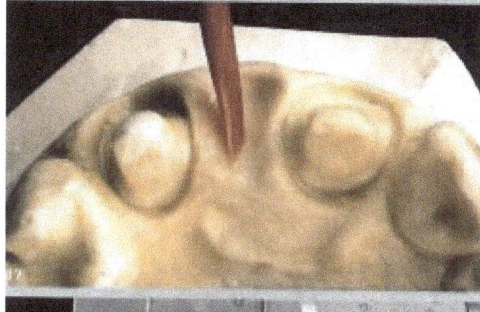

A separating medium (Multi-Sep, GC America) was applied to the abutments and surrounding structures of the stone model (Fig 17).

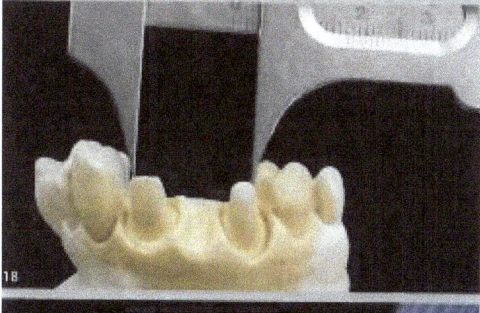

The distance between abutments was measured with a Boley gauge (Fig 18).

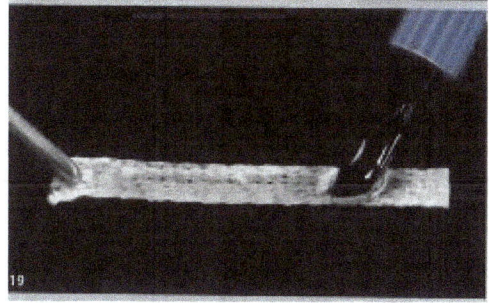

A plasma-coated reinforcement fiber 2 mm in width (Ribbond-THM, Rib-bond) was measured from this inter abutment dimension and coated with an unfilled light-cured resin-bonding adhesive (D/E Resin, Bisco) (Fig 19). The excess adhesive can be absorbed using a 2 x 2 lint-free gauze. The adhesive was light cured for 20 seconds

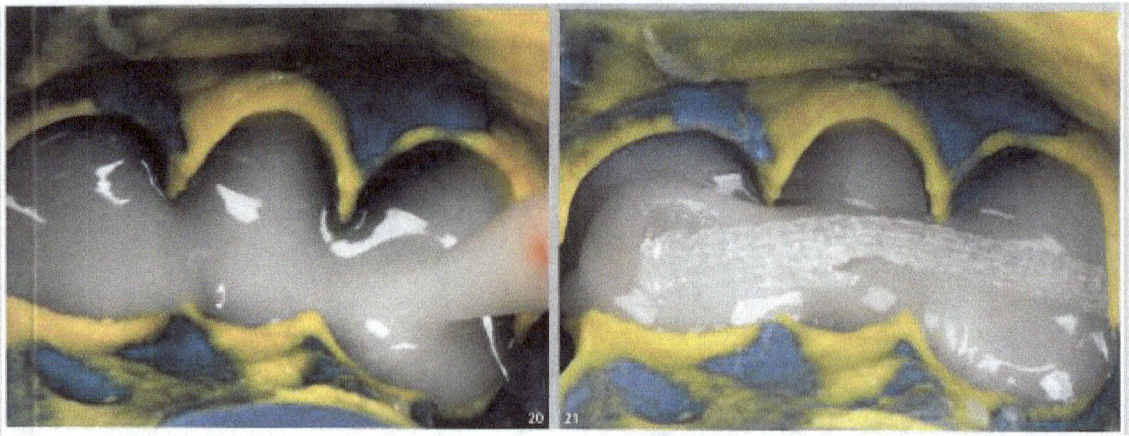

A bis-acryl provisional material (Luxatemp) was injected into the polyvinyl siloxane impression transfer lining the facial and lingual aspects of the impression in the region of the three-unit FPD. The pre-measured reinforcement fiber was immediately placed in the resin material (Fig 20 and 21).

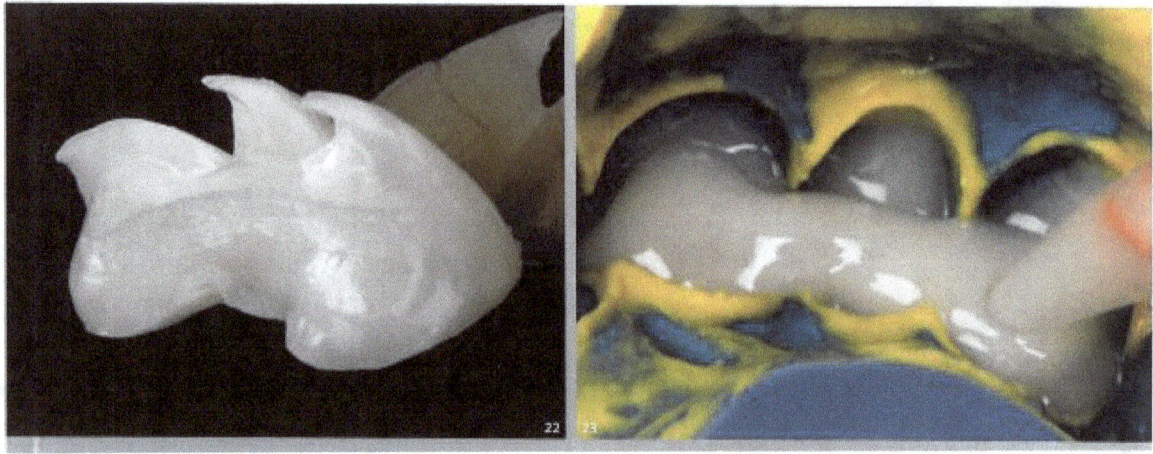

This cross-sectional photograph illustrates the position of the reinforcement fiber (Fig 22). A higher-chroma-shaded bis-acryl provisional material was injected over the reinforcement fiber as an "artificial dentin" core. (Fig 23).

PROVISIONALIZATION

DIRECT FABRICATION OF AN ANTERIOR PROVISIONAL CROWN

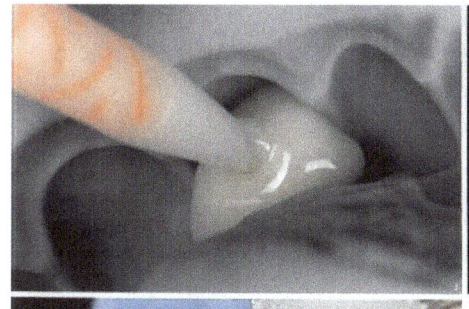
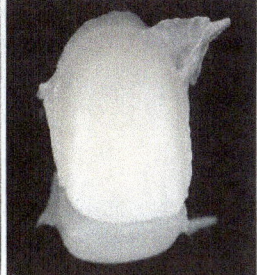
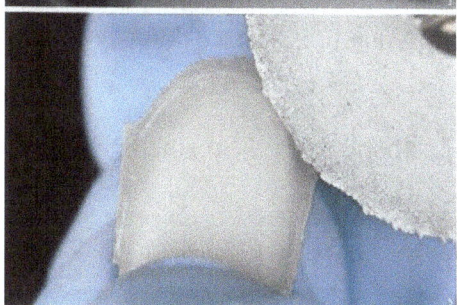

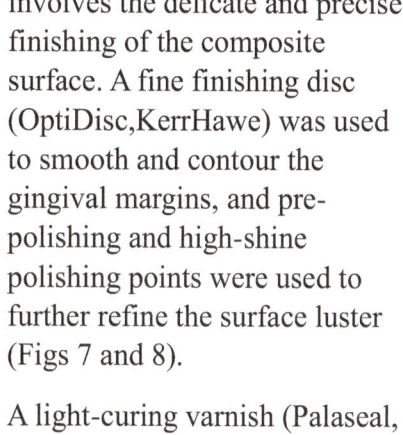

FIGURE 8.3: Fine finishing involves the delicate and precise finishing of the composite surface. A fine finishing disc (OptiDisc, KerrHawe) was used to smooth and contour the gingival margins, and pre-polishing and high-shine polishing points were used to further refine the surface luster (Figs 7 and 8).

A light-curing varnish (Palaseal, Heraeus Kulzer) was applied to the facial and lingual surfaces and polymerized for 60 seconds on each surface (Fig 9).

The interim restoration has become an integral component in the development and management of the design of the definitive prosthetic restoration. The only difference between the provisional and the definitive restoration should be the material from which it is made (Figs 10 to 14)

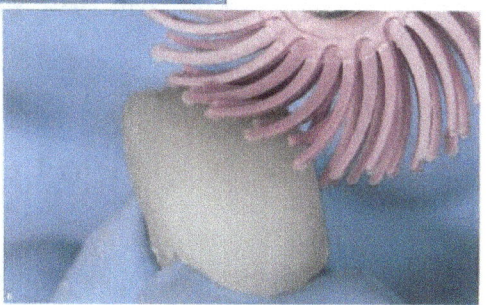

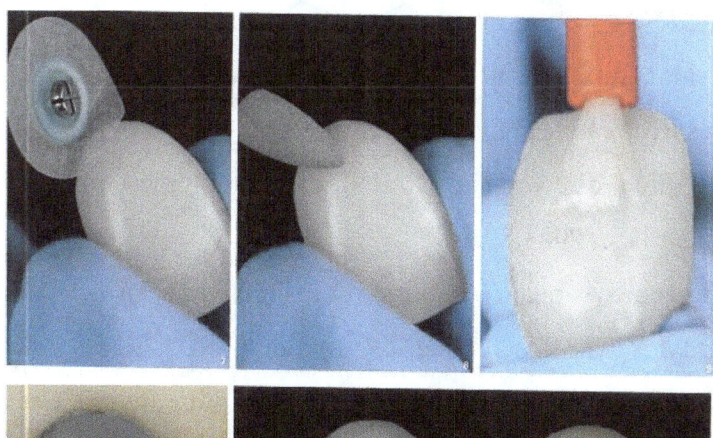

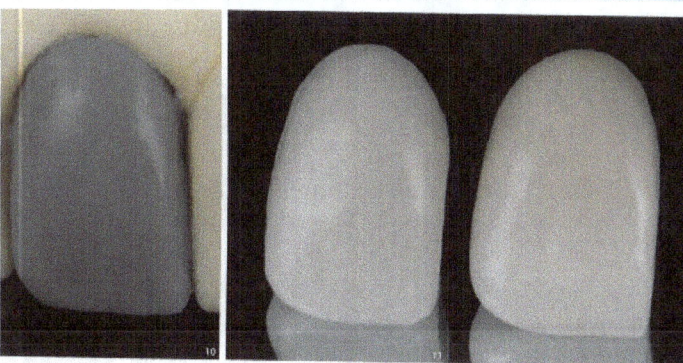

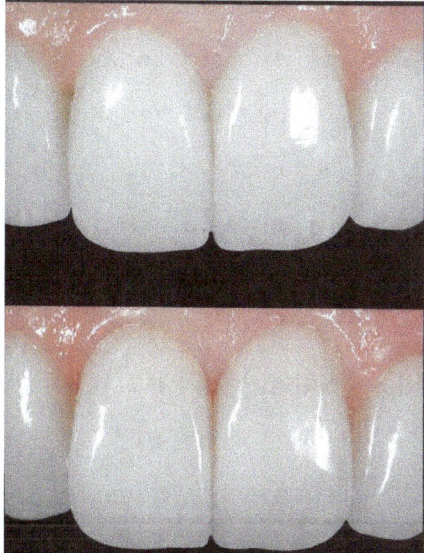

118 | Page

REFERENCES

1. **Terry DA.** The interim restoration. Pract Proced Aesthet Dent 2005; 17:263-264.
2. **Solow RA.** Composite veneered acrylic resin provisional restorations for complete veneer crowns. J Prosthet Dent 1999; 82:515-517.
3. **Albino JE, Tedesco LA, Conny DJ.** Patient perceptions of dental-facial esthetics: Shared concerns in orthodontics and prosthodontics. J Prosthet Dent 1985;53:451-454.
4. **Donovan T, Cho G.** Diagnostic provisional restorations in restorative dentistry: The blueprint for success. J Can Dent Assoc 1999; 65:272-275.
5. **Preston JD.** A systemic approach to the control of esthetic form. J Prosthet Dent 1976; 35:393-402.
6. **Yuodelis RA, Faucher R.** Provisional restorations: An integrated approach to periodontics and restorative dentistry. Dent Clin North Am 1980; 24:285-303.
7. **Saba S.** Anatomically correct soft tissue profiles using fixed detachable provisional im- plant restorations. J Can Dent Assoc 1997; 63:767-770.
8. **Cho GC, Chee WW.** Custom characterization of the provisional restoration. J Prosthet Dent 1993; 69:529-532.
9. **Cibirka RM, Linebaugh ML.** The fixed/detachable implant provisional prosthesis. J Pros- thodont 1997; 6:149-152.
10. **Rieder CE.** The use of provisional restorations to develop and achieve esthetic expectations.Int J Periodontics Restorative Dent 1989;9:123-139.
11. **Dumbrigue HB.** Composite indirect-direct method for fabricating multiple-unit provisional restorations. Prosthet Dent 2003;89:86-88.
12. **Fehling AW, Neitzke C.** A direct provisional restoration for decreased occlusal wear and improved marginal integrity: A hybrid technique. J Prosthodont 1994; 3:256-260.
13. **Boberick KG, Bachstein TK.** 1998 Judson C. Hickey Scientific Writing Award. Use of a flexible cast for the indirect fabrication of provisional restorations. J Prosthet Dent 1999; 82:90-93.
14. **Shillingburg HT Jr,Sather DA,Wilson EL Jr,et al.** Fundamentals of Fixed Prosthodontics, ed 4. Chicago: Quintessence,2012:241-243.
15. **Hamza TA, Rosenstiel SF, Elhosary MM, Ibraheem RM.** The effect of fiber reinforcement on the fracture toughness and flexural strength of provisional restorative resins. J Prosthet Dent 2004; 91:258-264.

16. **Krug RS.** Temporary resin crowns and bridges. Dent Clin North Am 1975; 19:313-320.
17. **Vahidi F.** The provisional restoration. Dent Clin North Am 1987; 31:363-381.
18. **Cleveland JL Jr, Richardson JT.** Surface characterization of temporary restorations: Guidelines for quality ceramics. J Prosthet Dent 1977; 37:643-647.
19. **Nixon RL.** Provisionalization for ceramic laminate veneer restorations: A clinical update. Pract Periodontics Aesthet Dent 1997; 9:17-28.
20. **Galindo D, Soltys JL, Graser GN.** Long-term reinforced fixed provisional restorations. J Pros-thet Dent 1998; 79:698-701.
21. **Dykema RW, Goodacre CJ, Phillips RW.** Johnston's Modern Practice in Fixed Prosthodontics, ed 4. St Louis: WB Saunders, 1986:77-90.
22. **Amsterdam M, Fox L.** Provisional splinting—Principles and techniques. Dent Clin North Am 1959; 1:73-99.
23. **Antonelli JR, Gulker I.** A modified indirect working die technique for fabricating provisional restorations for multiple teeth. Quintessence Int 2000; 31:392-396.
24. **Nemcovsky E, Gross MD.** Transferring provisional restorations to final master casts. J Oral Rehabil 1994; 21:157-163.
25. **Bral M.** Periodontal considerations for provisional restorations. Dent Clin North Am 1989; 33:457-476.
26. **Fox CW, Abrams BL, Doukoudakis A.** Provisional restorations for altered occlusions. J Pros-thet Dent 1984; 52:567-572.
27. **Liebenberg WH.** Multiple porcelain veneers: A temporization innovation—The peripheral seal technique. J Can Dent Assoc 1996; 62:70-78.
28. **Federick DR.** The provisional fixed partial denture. J Prosthet Dent 1975; 34:520-526.
29. **Davidoff SR.** Heat-processed acrylic resin provisional restorations: An in-office procedure. J Prosthet Dent 1982; 48:673-675
30. **Nayer A, Edwards WS.** Fabrication of a single anterior intermediate restoration. J Prosthet Dent 1978; 39:574-577.
31. **Gennaro RL Jr.** The injection-molded technique for anterior maxillary provisional restorations: A clinical case. Pract Proced Aesthet Dent 2002; 14:251-256.
32. **Zalkind M, Flochman N.** Laminate veneer provisional restorations: A clinical report. J Prosthet Dent 1997; 77:109-110.

33. **Elledge DA, Hart JK, Schorr BL.** A provisional restoration technique for laminate veneer preparations. J Prosthet Dent 1989; 62:139-142.
34. **Dumfahrt FI, Gobel G.** Bonding porcelain laminate veneer provisional restorations: An experimental study. J Prosthet Dent 1999; 82:281-285.
35. **Bennani V.** Fabrication of an indirect-direct provisional fixed partial denture. J Prosthet Dent 2000; 84:364-365.
36. **Gurel G.** The Science and Art of Porcelain Laminate Veneers. Berlin: Quintessence, 2003. 119.
37. **Gurel G, Bichacho N.** Permanent diagnostic provisional restorations for predictable results when redesigning the smile. Pract Proced Aesthet Dent 2006; 18:281-317.
38. **Wassell RW, St George G, Ingledew RP, Steele JG.** Crowns and other extra-coronal restorations: Provisional restorations. Br Dent J 2002; 192:619-630.
39. **Wood M, Halpern BG, Lamb MF.** Visible light-cured composite resins: An alternative for anterior provisional restorations. J Prosthet Dent 1984; 51:192-194.
40. **Sadan A.** Clinical considerations in cement selection for provisional restorations— Part I. Pract Periodontics Aesthet Dent 2000; 12:638.

CHAPTER-10

FINISHING AND POLISHING

Restorative materials of the past such as amalgam and gold required finishing and polishing procedures to refine anatomical morphology, contours, marginal integrity, and occlusion while enhancing the surface smoothness of the restorations. The objectives of finishing and polishing techniques of tooth-colored restorations are the same today, except that the development of tooth-colored restorative materials has introduced a new element in the restorative equation—esthetics. The objective of esthetic restorative dentistry has become one of achieving and displaying restorations of beautiful, natural-looking teeth that will maintain function and assure the structural integrity of the teeth while eliminating the appearance of metal such as gold and amalgam during smiling or phonation.[1] An optimally finished esthetic adhesive restoration should provide a smooth surface that will prevent plaque accumulation[2-6] and resist staining.[7] It should also possess ideal contours and an emergence profile for improved tissue compatibility.[7] Additional benefits of a proper finish are anatomical form for occlusal harmony,[7] shade coordination to surrounding dentition,[7] symmetric surface texture to adjacent or opposing natural teeth, improved marginal adaptation and integrity,[7-8] longevity, and esthetics.[6,8,9]

In general, finishing focuses on contouring, adjusting, shaping, and smoothing the restoration to obtain desired anatomy, while polishing concentrates on producing a smooth surface luster and highly light-reflective surface.[10] The technique for removal or trimming of composite resin or porcelain can be developed in three sequential steps: contouring, fine finishing, and polishing. Contouring involves the gross reduction of the composite or ceramic restoration to obtain the desired form and shape as determined by the parameters of function and esthetic considerations.[11] Fine finishing comprises the delicate and precise finishing of the margins, removing surface defects and scratches and developing a smoother surface.[9] Polishing consists of reducing the roughness and scratches produced during the finishing procedure.[12]

During the polishing procedure, the objective is to reduce the surface irregularities so that the distance between the scratches is less than the wavelength of visible light (approximately 0.5 pm), making the surface as reflective as enamel.[13] A surface appears smooth when its roughness is significantly less than 1 pm.[14-15] These procedural steps should be performed in sequence using abrasives in various types of devices. The principle is similar to metal polishing, in which the sequence of abrasives progresses from the coarsest abrasive to the finest.[16] The abrasiveness of one particle or material against another depends on its hardness.[17]

Hardness has been defined as the resistance to permanent indentation or penetration.[12] In order for a finishing and polishing system to be effective, the cutting particles (abrasives) must be harder than the filler component of the restorative material.[18-19] Accordingly, the effectiveness of the finishing and polishing process depends on the type of restorative material utilized. Various types of hand and rotary instruments and finishing and polishing devices utilizing assorted wet and dry techniques have been advocated for and argued about by technicians and clinicians. A multitude of finishing and polishing devices are available to the laboratory technician and restorative dentist, including multi-fluted carbide burs, micron-sized finishing diamonds, silicon carbide-coated and aluminum oxide-coated abrasive discs, abrasive white and green stones, abrasive strips, light-cured resin points, and impregnated-rubber or silicone discs, wheels, points, cups, and polishing pastes.[9, 12, 20, 21] While no demonstrable statistical difference exists between finishing and polishing anterior and posterior restorative materials,[22] the consideration factors for finishing and polishing any restoration are dependent on the instrument shape, the tooth and restoration surface shape and texture, the surface of finishing and polishing instruments, and the sequence of the restorative treatment.[7-22] Successful finishing and polishing of any restoration is determined by the type of restorative material used (composition and structure of the material) and the shape of the finishing device and defined by the surface morphology of the tooth and restoration. Because the geometry and shape of the natural teeth and these devices essentially remain the same over time, the only variable is the continual change in the formulation of the restorative material.

CLASSIFICATION OF ABRASIVES

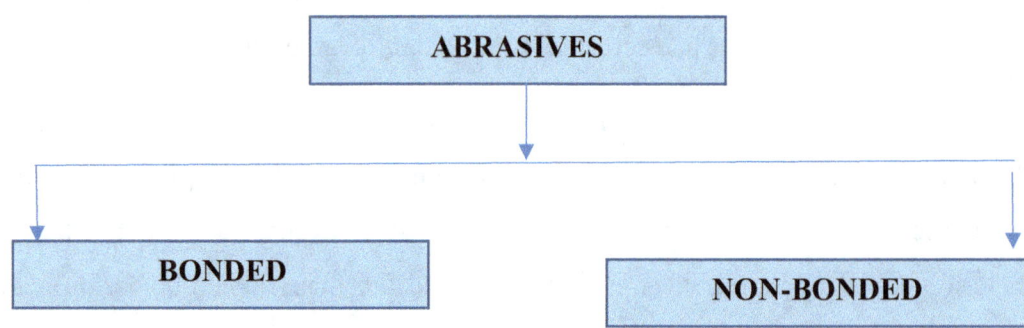

FINISHING AND POLISHING

BASED ON GRITS

- **COARSE** (125-150 um)
- **MEDIUM COARSE** (90-100 um)
- **MEDIUM FINE** (88-125um)
- **FINE** (60-74um)
- **SUPER FINE** (38-44um)

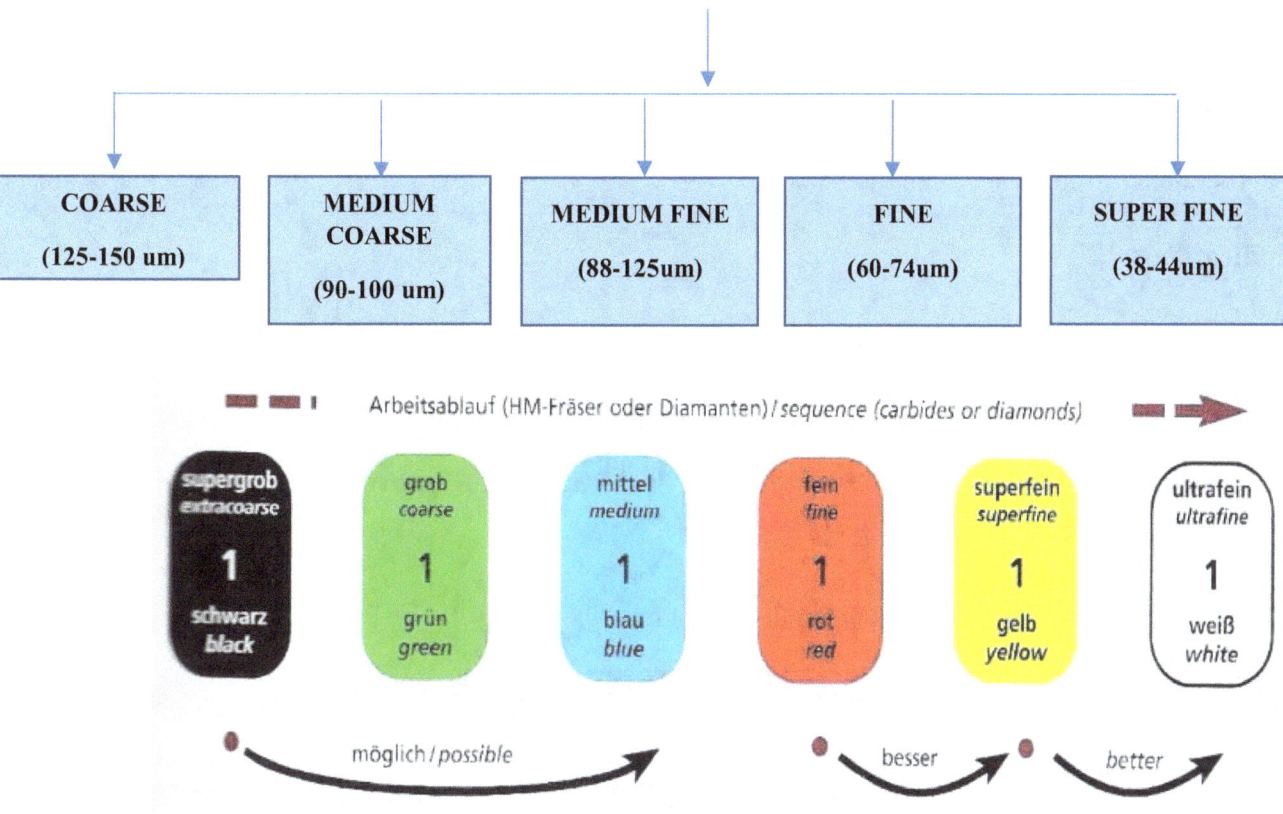

FIG 10.1: COLOUR CODING OF BURS

CLASSIFICATION OF FINISHING AND POLISHING INSTRUMENTS

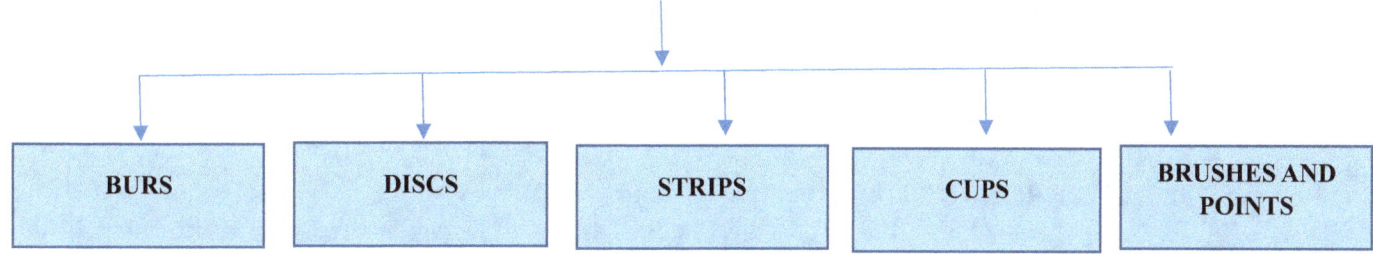

- BURS
- DISCS
- STRIPS
- CUPS
- BRUSHES AND POINTS

SUPER-SNAP RAINBOW KIT

A comprehensive, color-coded, disposable disc/poly strip system for composite finishing and polishing.

Benefits:

• Discs are extremely thin and highly flexible

• No metal center

• Consistent 4-step contouring, finishing, and polishing & Super polishing system

- Coordinated polishing strips for interproximal areas
- No gouging of enamel or restoration
- Secure hold of the disk onto the mandrel (maximum control during polishing)
- Disk come in 12mm and 8mm diameter

Indications:

For Contouring, finishing, polishing, and super polishing of Anterior composite restorations

- Contouring: Super-Snap disk black (coarse).
- Finishing: Super-Snap disk violet (medium • Polishing: Super-Snap disk green (fine) • Super polishing: Super-Snap disk Red (superfine)
- For interproximal finishing and polishing use Super Snap Poly strips.

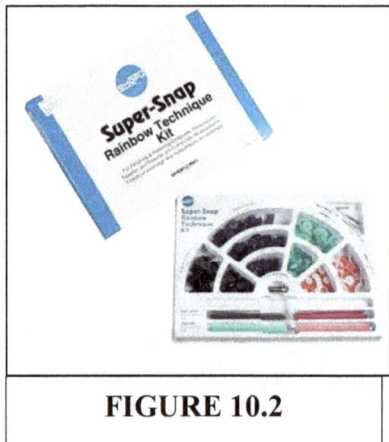

FIGURE 10.2

SUPER SNAP POLY STRIPS

Polyester Strips for contouring, finishing, polishing and super polishing inter proximal areas of composite restorations

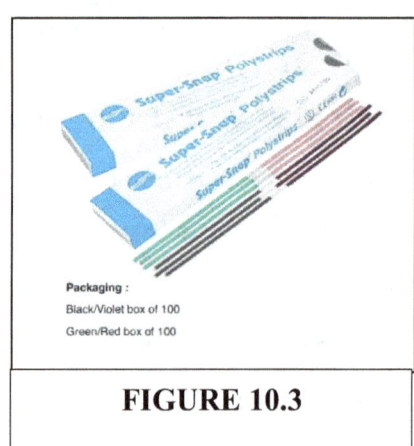

FIGURE 10.3

FINISHING AND POLISHING

ONE GLOSS SET

One-stop solution for finishing & polishing direct restorations

Benefits:

• Aluminium Oxide impregnated Silicone points provide Optimal Abrasive Performance

• Finishing & Polishing with only one Instrument just by altering the Contact Pressure (Friction)

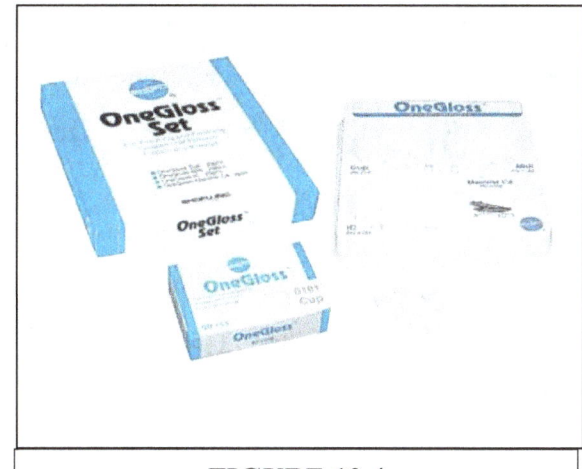

FIGURE 10.4

• Eliminates the need for Polishing Paste • Low Vibrations and minimal Heat Generation

Indications:

• For Finishing and Polishing Composite and glass-ionomer restorations

• For removal of excess cement without marring delicate inlays, as well as for the removal of Surface stains

• After orthodontic bracket debonding in order to remove the excess bonded cement without decalcifying the enamel

• Polishing of enamel after scaling

• Creating Surface textures on direct cosmetic restorations

SUPER-SNAP BUFF DISC

Buffing is an important part of abrasive procedures and involves the production of Micro Fine scratches over the restoration thus producing extra lustre and enhancing the overall composure of the restoration.

Benefits:

• Felt disc retains polishing paste with minimum splatter or wastage during use

• Requires feather light touch to produce a high gloss polish

• Flexible yet resilient discs easily adapt to the natural contours of the tooth surface

• Absence of metal center or exposed mandrel prevents gouging or discoloration of Tooth/Restoration • Available in 2 sizes: 12mm & 8mm

Indications:

Specially designed buff disc made of synthetic felt polishing cloth for buffing of

• Composites,

• Porcelain,

• Acrylic Teeth and

• Gold Restorations

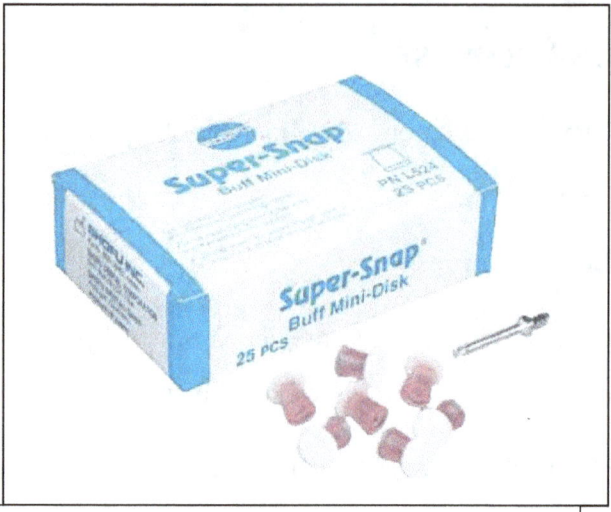

FIGURE 10.5

COMPOSITE FINISHING KIT CA/FG

Concise kit with assorted stones for precise finishing of direct composite and glass ionomer restorations

Benefits:

• Consists of coarse dura green (silicone carbide) stones for contouring and fine dura white (aluminium oxide) stones for finer finishing.

• Available in both contra-angled handpiece mandrel (CA) & airotor mandrel (FG

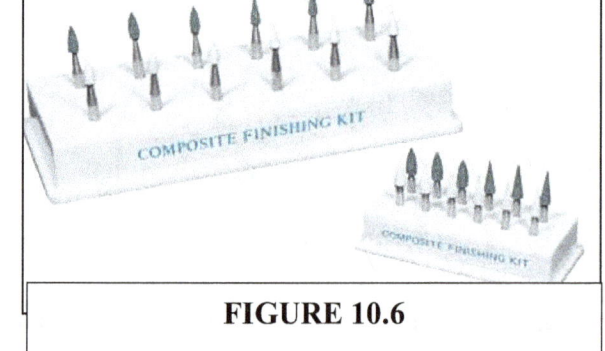

FIGURE 10.6

• Autoclavable stones which are durable and long-lasting

Indications: Designed for contouring and finishing direct resin and glass ionomer restorations

COMPOSITE POLISHING KIT CA

Benefits:

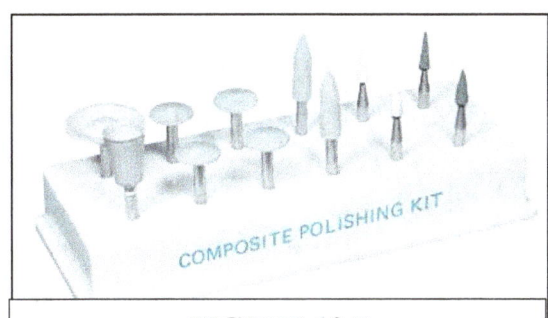

- The durable abrasive points are autoclavable and cost-effective

- Comprehensive selection of points for finishing and polishing in one kit

FIGURE 10.7

- For fast and efficient finishing the use of composite finishing kit FG is recommended in conjunction with the composite polishing kit

Indications: Comprehensive assortment of finishing and polishing of direct resins and glass ionomers.

COMPOMASTER ASSORTMENT

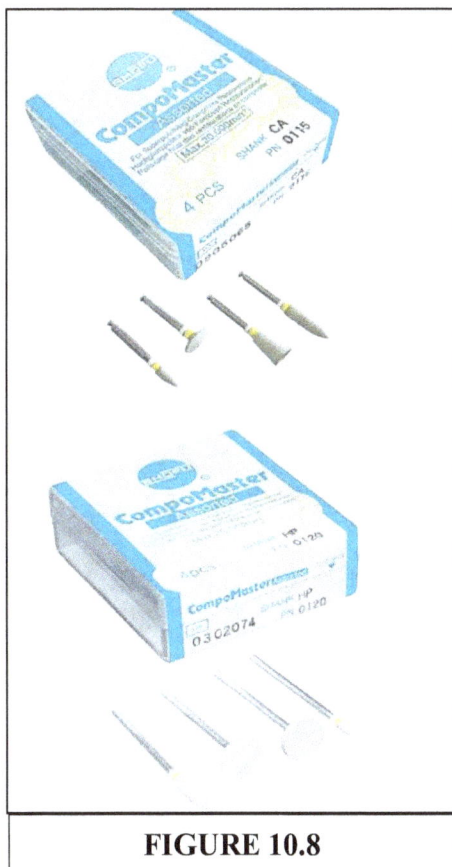

Advanced diamond-impregnated abrasive system for enhanced finishing, pre-polishing & super-polishing of composite restorations

CompoMaster Coarse (yellow polisher) - For finishing & basic polishing

CompoMaster Regular (yellow & white bands) - For super polishing

Indications: High-end polishing of direct & indirect composite restorations

FIGURE 10.8

CERAMAGE POLISHING KIT

SPECIALLY DESIGNED FOR SYSTEMATIC POLISHING OF INDIRECT COMPOSITES

A careful selection of trimming, finishing, and polishing instruments for a precise functional and aesthetic enhancement of indirect composites. (CERAMAGE)

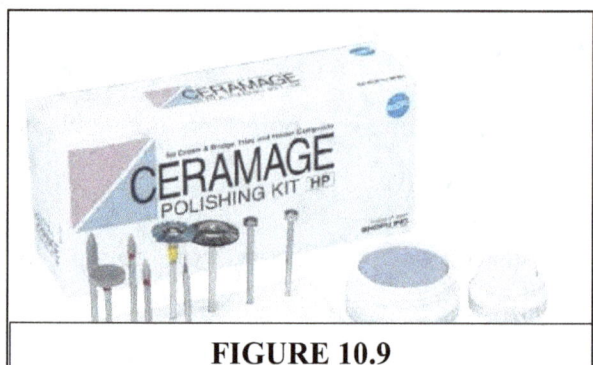

FIGURE 10.9

REFERENCES

1. **Touati B.** Bonded ceramic restorations: Achieving predictability. Pract Periodontics Aes- that Dent 1995; 7:33-37.

2. **Stewart GP, Bachman TA, Hatton JF.** Temperature rise due to finishing of direct restorative materials. Am J Dent 1991; 4:23-28.

3. **Cooley RL, Barkmeier WW, White JH.** Heat generation during polishing of restorations. Quintessence Int Dent Dig 1978;9(12):77-80.

4. **Bollen CM, Lambrechts P, Quirynen M.** Comparison of surface roughness of oral hard materials to the threshold surface roughness for bacterial plaque retention: A review of the literature. Dent Mater 1997; 13:258-269.

5. **Kaplan BA, Goldstein GR, Vijayaraghavan TV, Nelson IK.** The effect of three polishing systems on the surface roughness of four hybrid composites: A profilometric and scanning electron microscopy study. J Proshet Dent 1996; 76:34-38.

6. **Berastegui E, Canalda C, Brau E, Miquel C.** Surface roughness of finished composite resin. J Prosthet Dent 1992; 68:742-749.

7. **Goldstein RE.** Finishing of composites and laminates. Dent Clin North Am 1989; 33:305-318.

8. **Yap AU, Ang HQ, Chong KC.** Influence of finishing time on marginal sealing ability of new generation composite bonding systems. J Oral Rehabil 1998; 25:871-876.

9. **Jefferies SR.** The art and science of abrasive finishing and polishing in restorative dentistry. Dent Clin North Am 1998; 42:613-627.

10. **Summitt JB, Robbins JW, Hilton TJ, Schwartz RS.** Finishing and polishing. In: Fundamentals of Operative Dentistry: A Contemporary Approach. Chicago: Quintessence,1996:201-205.

11. **Lutz F, Setcos JC, Phillips RW.** New finishing instruments for composite resins. J Am Dent Assoc 1983; 107:575-580.

12. **Yap AU, Sau CW, Lye KW.** Effects of finishing/polishing time on surface characteristics of tooth-colored restoratives. J Oral Rehabil 1998; 25:456-461.

13. **Van Noort R.** Controversial aspects of composite resin restorative materials. Br Dent J 1983; 155:380-385.

14. **Chung KH.** Effects of finishing and polishing procedures on the surface texture of resin composites. Dent Mater 1994; 10:325-330.

15. **Jung M.** Finishing and polishing of a hybrid composite and a heat-pressed glass ceramic. Oper Dent 2002; 27:175-183.
16. **Strassler HE.** Polishing composite resins. J Esthet Dent 1992; 4:177-179.
17. **Mitchell CA, Pintado MR, Douglas WH.** Iatrogenic tooth abrasion comparisons among composite materials and finishing techniques. J Prosthet Dent 2002; 88:320-328.
18. **Chandler HH, Bowen RL, Paffenbarger GC.** Method for finishing composite restorative materials. J Am Dent Assoc 1971; 83:344-348.
19. **Tjan AH, Chan CA.** The polishability of posterior composites. J Prosthet Dent 1989;61:138-146.
20. **Horton CB, Paules HM, Pelleu GB, Rudolph JJ.** An evaluation of commercial pastes for finishing composite resin surfaces. J Prosthet Dent 1977; 37:674-679.
21. **Toledano M, De La Torre FJ, Osorio R.** Evaluation of two polishing methods for resin composites. Am J Dent 1994; 7:328-330.
22. **Pratten DH, Johnson GH.** An evaluation of finishing instruments for an anterior and a posterior composite. J Prosthet Dent 1988; 60:154-158.
23. Final-SDI-Clinical-Catalog-2019-Folder_compressed.pdf (shofu.co.in)

www.ingramcontent.com/pod-product-compliance
Lightning Source LLC
Chambersburg PA
CBHW062217220526
45471CB00009B/3235